D0341768

Tested By Fire

Tested By Fire

by Merrill and Virginia Womach
with Mel and Lyla White

Fleming H. Revell Company
Old Tappan, New Jersey

Scripture quotations are from the King James Version of the Bible.

Library of Congress Cataloging in Publication Data

Womach, Virginia.
  Tested by fire.

  1. Womach, Merrill. 2. Womach, Virginia.
I. Womach, Merrill, joint author. II. White, Mel,
joint author. III. White, Lyla, joint author.
IV. Title.
BR1725.W595W65   248'.2'0924 [B]   75-42789
ISBN 0-8007-0782-6

TO Virginia—who never stopped loving me
TO Merrill—whose courage was contagious
TO our beloved children—who shared of their
strength in our hour of need
and
TO our Lord—a never-failing Friend in
time of trouble

Contents

Tested By Fire

1

All I Could See Was Fire

THE SKIES ABOVE LOS ANGELES were dark at midday. A hard rain slowed freeway traffic to a snail's pace. Visibility was decreasing rapidly. Any moment the airport would close and leave me stranded twelve hundred miles from Spokane, Washington, and our family's annual Thanksgiving Day reunion. At last my driver turned onto the field and helped me load my records and recording equipment into the blue and white, four-seat Piper Apache waiting there.

"Aren't you afraid to fly in this kind of weather?" he asked.

"No," I answered glibly. "After all, if I go down, I'll go down singing."

It was a bad joke, and ominous as the storm front that covered the West Coast from San Diego to Seattle. The tower cleared takeoff and moments later I was airborne.

Tomorrow was Thanksgiving. My mother would sit at the head of a long festive table in our old family home, welcoming sons, daughters, in-laws, and grandchildren to that annual feast. Dad would say grace, his eyes filled with grateful tears to have his family home again. I had not missed a reunion in thirty-four years and refused to let the weather keep me from this one. Besides, my wife and three young children had spent too much time alone in the past years, as I flew around the country building our new business and singing before church groups, service clubs, and school assemblies. I suppose it was as much guilt as courage that got me up that day.

* * * * *

I SHARED MERRILL'S DREAM. One day our National Music Service Company would provide quality music systems to funeral homes across America. With our growing staff and rising costs, he had no choice but to fly up and down the country demonstrating, installing, and servicing as many accounts as possible.

Still, I hated those long, lonely nights without him. Our house creaks and moans and rattles when he is gone, and is perfectly silent when he is home again. So when I am alone at night I sleep with a machete under the bed. We once used it as a Roman sword in a church Easter play, and although I can't imagine using it for protection, there is some comfort in having it there. One night Merrill came home from a trip earlier than I expected. Not wanting to awaken me, he entered quietly without turning on the lights and began going over his mail on the kitchen counter top. Thinking him a burglar, I sneaked up behind him with my machete, yelled loudly, and scared him right back out into the street again.

The day before that fateful Thanksgiving he called me from the airport in Klamath Falls, Oregon. "I will be home tonight," he said, "on two conditions—first, if the weather doesn't get any worse, and second, if you promise not to attack me with your machete."

* * * * *

I DIDN'T TELL VIRGINIA in that call how bad the weather was or that I had already tried once to beat the storm out of Klamath Falls and was forced back to the field by strong winds and snow flurries. After hearing her voice, I determined to try again. In the coffee shop I sat next to a young pilot who had been forced down at Klamath Falls just after I had. His teeth were chattering. His hand shook so wildly that coffee sloshed out of his cup and splashed against the table.

"Pretty bad up there," I mentioned casually, "but I think I'll try it again."

"Are you kidding?" he answered. "I hit winds so rough that one downdraft sent my heavy briefcase spiraling from one side of the plane, knocking out the window on the opposite side and disappearing into the storm."

His warning should have stopped me from flying, but a man this close to home is difficult to persuade. I stayed on the ground for about three hours and then took off to the north, following Highway 97 up around Klamath Lake. The weather was bad. Large wet snowflakes began falling again as I descended to the minimum altitude. I didn't have my instrument rating then and had to fly by visual flight rules. Under VFR you have to follow the reference to the ground—roads, trees, towns—anything that helps you get your bearings.

The snow was falling faster. There was an emergency landing strip right off the road—if I could keep going long enough. Those can be famous last words to a pilot in too big a hurry. I was flying where I should not have been. And I was trapped. I felt as though I was in one of those old-fashioned round paperweights filled with fake snow. When you turn it upside down and shake it, you create a blizzard. I was inside the blizzard trying to see out.

My ground references were obliterated in a blanket of white. The windshields were panels of frost and slush. I was losing my bearings. Up and down, land and sky all merged into one, when suddenly just below me I saw the emergency strip near Beaver Marsh, Oregon. The little orange pylons stood out in a world of white and I nosed down between them with a great sigh of gratitude and relief.

* * * * *

WHEN MERRILL CALLED from Beaver Marsh I had no idea of the horror he had just escaped or the tragedy that lay ahead. On the road he calls only to reassure me, in spite of what he is going through.

"I will be late, honey. It is snowing and I am going to wait it out at Beaver Marsh. But I will fly in on Thanksgiving morning and make it for the reunion. Don't worry."

"Stay warm," I advised him, "and don't take any chances." It was not a conversation, really; it was a routine by now. Husband reassuring wife, wife receiving message. Over and out. After all, he had flown fifteen hundred hours in all kinds of airplanes without incident, and during those same hours I had tended our children without loss. So we did not really need to communicate, just check in. I was capable wife, cook, business partner, keeper of the house, and he was successful man-on-the-go. We loved each other, but our communications had been reduced to signals.

"I am going to be late," he signalled.

"Stay warm," I signalled back.

Then silence. I hung up the phone, my mind whirling with what I wanted to tell him. "I love you, Merrill. Come home—I'm afraid." Instead, I turned back to Dan and Marlene and Judie. Dan, our nine-year-old son, was trying gamely to cut out pie crusts. Marlene, fourteen, was mashing sweet potatoes, and Judie, sixteen, was mixing in the brown sugar, butter, and honey. The room was quiet. Thanksgiving dinner smells filled the room. I walked over to the children and began putting the sweet potatoes into the little pastry bag, and squeezing them into flower designs complete with marshmallow tops before baking.

"Daddy is okay," I signalled the family.

"Good," they signalled back. And down inside me was a growing urge to hold Merrill and the children safely in my arms and cry for all we were not saying to each other.

*   *   *   *   *

BEAVER MARSH is an emergency landing strip, an A-frame motel, a service station, and a coffee shop with a few homes and house trailers clustered about. Highway 97 is its front porch, its entertainment, its view on the world. The people who live in Beaver Marsh are there to service the highway and its millions of motorists who speed by, never noticing Beaver Marsh or the people who live there.

In the silence of that snowstorm, Beaver Marsh felt isolated and abandoned. I taxied to the parking area, shut down the two 150-horsepower engines which had carried me safely through that storm, took out my traveling kit, and walked to the motel.

"Any rooms?" I asked the clerk who must have heard me land.

"Every one of them," he smiled back.

After a meal at the coffee shop, I returned to the motel and struck up a conversation with the owner. When he learned I was a musician, he invited me to play the organ in their living quarters. I sang and played only one song before he disappeared into the kitchen. I could hear him on the phone inviting all of Beaver Marsh to an impromptu concert that apparently I was about to perform. In minutes the coffee shop was closed, the service station was locked, and the people of Beaver Marsh were crowded into that living room listening to old gospel songs, laughing and crying and making requests, singing spirituals, and enjoying each other.

It was one of those incredible moments when the unexpected draws people together. Piles of new-fallen snow blocked the highway running between them. Unable to continue the tasks that usually kept them apart, the people turned to each other. For those moments they were again a community of friends, a family. They came in out of the storm, sat side by side, drank coffee, talked, touched, made jokes, sang—"Sweet hour of prayer! Sweet hour of prayer! That calls me from a world of care"—and disappeared back into the storm again.

I was tired long before they were, but kept playing and singing until after midnight. I went to sleep the moment my head touched that damp, stiffly starched motel pillow. In the morning there was no hot water in the place and I had to use my double-edged razor with cold water. I remember muttering complaints all the time I was shaving. It was the last time I would ever shave.

I joined three men whom I had met the night before having morning coffee at the cafe. We talked for a long time. I suppose it was my reluctance to get back in the air. The clouds were not very high and there was a lot of snow and slush and ice. I called the Weather Bureau and found that the weather was passable up north. Since that Thanksgiving reunion was only hours away, I paid my bill and said good-by to these new though nameless friends. Twenty minutes later they would save my life.

I started the engines, went through my pre-takeoff checklist, taxied to the end of the landing strip, and took off to the south. There was no indication of trouble ahead. The clouds were quite high. Visibility was increasing. I was about three hundred feet above the trees and the plane was responding normally when, without any warning, both engines quit. Apparently the snow and icy slush on the runway had packed itself against the air induction intakes on the engines. When I got above the height of the trees, this snow and slush froze in place and starved the engines of their needed oxygen. So they stopped. I had to land immediately.

Ahead of me was a forest of sturdy Oregon timber. Already I was losing altitude, but I did not want to tangle with those trees. I could land on Highway 97 below me, but the road was filled with drivers anxious to make up for time lost in the storm. A large blue truck-and-trailer rig, several automobiles, and a camper were directly in my path. I couldn't risk crashing into any one or all of these.

So I made the next best decision and tried to make a 180-degree turn to get back to the runway. The trees rushed up at me. The airplane began to shake. I knew it would stall and fall at any moment. I hoped to keep the plane up through sheer willpower and strained to make that long turn to safety.

One hundred and fifty yards from the end of the runway I hit the first tree at about 85 miles per hour. That first blow knocked me unconscious. The plane whipped around and plunged tail first through those trees for another 100 yards. Upon final impact, 108 gallons of gasoline exploded and I awoke in a sea of flames, 50 yards from the runway.

When I first opened my eyes, I was sitting in the middle of a bonfire, surrounded by flames. All I could see was fire. I reached for the door with my right hand and tried to undo my safety belt with my left. The belt would not come free. I tore at it with both hands. Still the buckle held, its locking mechanism jammed by the impact. I remember very vividly taking that flameproof seat belt in my hands and ripping it in two. There is a perfectly reasonable explanation as to how a man in my condition could tear apart a 500-pound-test thick nylon belt. It is incredible to realize how God has made our bodies to respond in times of crisis. Adrenaline was the first miracle in a series of miracles that proved God's presence even in this fiery, painful experience.

I stumbled from the exploding plane and fell gasping into the snow. I crawled as quickly as I could from the burning wreckage. My plane, my recording equipment, my speaker system which I use in concerts, and my briefcase filled with important orders and contracts were all being consumed in a huge ball of flame.

I was not conscious of how seriously I had been burned. I was alive and it felt good to be stumbling toward the highway. But I could not see. That ball of fire seemed etched in my memory but no new picture would form. I ran into the trees. Long, low branches knocked me down and the heavy new snow fell on me, cooling my burns but disorienting me further. My flight became a nightmare of running, tripping, falling, getting up again. Branches like giant arms reached out to trap me and prevent my escape. Yet in the distance the noises from Highway 97 grew louder. I felt my way through the cold, wet darkness towards those sounds of life and rescue.

There was no way to know then, but help was on its way. Those same men in the coffee shop heard the engines die, and ran out to see my plane falling into the trees. They jumped into an old station wagon and drove rapidly to the scene. As I stumbled onto the highway they were there to catch me and place me in the backseat for the long ride to Klamath Falls and the only nearby hospital.

As I lay down an incredible thing happened. I was in horrible pain. My head and hands were completely burned. My eyes were swollen shut. I wanted to know what had happened to me, so I reached up and forced one eye open. Though blurred, I could see the skin on the back of my hands. It was charred like a bloody piece of steak that had slipped through the barbecue grill and onto the open fire. My hands looked ghastly. But instead of crying out in pain and horror and shock, I felt like singing.

The car door slammed. I could feel every bump as we moved from the rough shoulder onto Highway 97. My clothes were in shreds except for my synthetic jacket that had become hard as rock in the flames. My head was swelling and the pain grew more and more intense. Still I felt like singing. It was an old gospel song I had learned as a child. I don't know why that song came rushing out of me instead of cries of pain and pity, but it did.

The men drove and listened in disbelieving silence as out of the crack in my charcoal-broiled face came these old words:

> I've found the dear Saviour and now I'm made whole;
> I'm pardoned and have my release.
> His Spirit abiding and blessing my soul,
> Praise God, in my heart there is peace.*

At Collier State Park an ambulance met us and the attendants transferred me by stretcher and raced us away. They heard it, too, from my swollen, bleeding face:

Wonderful peace, Wonderful peace,
Peace that the world cannot give!
When I think how He brought me
From darkness to light,
There's a wonderful, wonderful peace.*

*From the song "Wonderful Peace" by Charles E. Braun. Copyright 1924. Renewed 1952 by Lillenas Publishing Co. Used by permission.

2

Don't Let That Man Be My Husband

MERRILL WAS OVERDUE. Three hours we had waited. Still no call from the airport, no cheery voice saying, "Come and get me." The first hour I didn't worry. It was snowing lightly in Spokane, but planes were flying. I had the children carefully wrap the sweet potatoes and the apple pies in foil. The ingredients for a giant salad were chilling in the refrigerator. The second hour we loaded everything into the car, including a fresh change of clothes for Merrill so we could go right from the airport to his parents' home across town. Finally, the phone rang.

"Hello, Virginia?" It wasn't his voice.

"Everyone is here but you and Merrill. Everything all right?" I stifled a sob. "Merrill hasn't called yet. I'm afraid something might be wrong."

The third hour we drove to the Womachs'. The sweet potatoes were getting colder. The pies were getting soggier and the giant salad was growing limp, but not nearly as limp as I had begun to feel. All thirty-four relatives greeted us. The table was set and waiting, but no one had the heart to begin the Thanksgiving feast without Merrill.

At first they tried to laugh and make jokes about the delay. Then the adults grew silent, puttering with the dinner or tending to the children. The younger ones played awhile, breaking into our gloom with squeals of laughter. Then, sensing something wrong, they too grew tense and fidgety. Finally, we decided to serve the dinner before it was spoiled completely by the delay.

Everyone ate nervously, one eye on the dinner, the other on the telephone. The food was hard for me to swallow. The waiting was becoming unbearable.

*   *   *   *   *

AS THE AMBULANCE ATTENDANTS wheeled me into that little country hospital, I had no idea how badly I had been burned. I could hear the doctor and the nurses clustered around my bed, but I could not see them. As they wrapped my legs, administered morphine and plasma, and cut away my asbestos-hard jacket, I asked for the telephone. One nurse held the phone to my lips while I tried to reach my family. I didn't want to frighten my wife or parents, so I called my brother Russell. By then my face had swollen to its limits. I could not move my lips. Fortunately, years before I had used a ventriloquist's dummy in my work as a youth pastor and I could speak without moving my lips.

*   *   *   *   *

WHEN THE PHONE FINALLY rang, everyone at the table jumped to answer it. We knew it would be Merrill.

"This is the operator. I have a person-to-person call for Russell Womach."

Russ left the table and went to the phone. Everyone waited for some word or gesture or look of surprise. All of us gathered around that phone, straining to catch some word of their conversation.

"I've had an accident," he said. "I'm in the hospital at Klamath Falls, but I am okay."

He talked as though he was not really hurt. He sounded natural. He admitted that he had been hurt somewhat but had gotten out without any broken bones. The plane had been destroyed. Some important records and equipment had been lost but he was fine.

When he hung up there was a unison sigh of relief, followed immediately by a flurry of phone calls. Trains were not available.

Planes were filled with holiday travelers. The bus had already gone for the day, and the snow made automobile travel dangerous and slow. But I had to see him. I had to know for myself that he was well.

Merrill's fellow workers in National Music Service, Wayne Town and Dwayne "Chris" Christensen, volunteered to drive me through the blizzard to Klamath Falls. Kathy Town made sandwiches to sustain us along the way. My parents came to take care of the children. Family and friends rallied to help me meet this crisis. Only those who have suffered can know how much those little acts of kindness can mean. They proved to me that a lot of people cared and it made those long, terrible days ahead easier to bear.

The children cried to go with us. They wanted to see their dad as badly as I did. But I assured them that they would see him in just a few days. I packed a small overnight case, thinking I would be back in Spokane with him in two or three days at most. Actually, I didn't get back to Spokane for two weeks, and the children didn't have their father back home again for three long months.

It took us seventeen hours to cover those 595 miles in the old Chevrolet van. The snow was falling heavily. Wind was whipping it into oversized drifts. Cars and trucks were in the ditch or flipped on their sides along the way. We had brought a sleeping bag, and one would drive, another would stare hopefully into the blizzard, and the third would try to sleep. The snowdrifts were almost impassable. No plows had gone before us. If it was smooth, we drove on it. We could not tell where the road was and where it wasn't.

When we finally arrived in Klamath Falls, a service-station attendant directed us to the emergency hospital. Discovering that old green apartment-house-turned-hospital was my first shock. The building was small, drab, and rundown. Paint was peeling in the corridors. There was a smell of death about the place. Inside the waiting room a small group of Indian men injured in a brawl were awaiting emergency aid. One young man had been knifed and was bleeding badly. Another sat holding his intestines in place with a towel covering an ugly stomach wound. Everyone was shouting and the young night nurse was doing her best to bring order in the chaos. She glanced up at me.

"My husband, Merrill Womach, is here. Could you tell me his room number, please?"

Her expression changed. She stood, spoke quickly, then walked away. "Please wait here, Mrs. Womach, until the doctor can see you."

An orderly led the two injured Indian boys away. I waited with growing alarm. Finally the doctor appeared. He looked haggard and harassed. The crowd of men circled him, asking questions about their injured friends. He worked his way through them and stood before me. He was not well suited for the task of preparing a wife to see what is left of the one she loves.

"Mrs. Womach, I want you to know that your husband will not look quite like himself. He has been slightly burned."

With that understatement to prepare me, he led me to a closet-like room where I was dressed in a nurse's gown and cap.

"Why the cap and gown to see a man who escaped a crash with no broken bones?" I thought to myself.

As we approached Merrill's room, I saw a basin of blood-red liquid and I almost fainted. "My word," I muttered, "he must be bleeding terribly."

"That's antiseptic solution to wash your hands, Mrs. Womach," he instructed me. "You must not carry infection to your husband."

As I washed my hands in the thick red solution, a feeling of dread began to grip me. I found it hard to breathe. I was walking in a dream. Then, out of the corner of one eye, I glimpsed a man lying on the bed inside. He was horribly burned. His head was swollen larger than a basketball. Flesh hung in dark black folds. His hands were bleeding, black, and ugly.

"Dear God," I whispered, "don't let that man be my husband."
Then he spoke.

"Is someone there?"

It was Merrill's voice coming out of that burned, bleeding face.

"Yes, honey, I'm here." Swallowing hard to breathe and struggling to maintain composure, I went over to him and patted him on the shoulder. His head looked like a marshmallow that had been put into a fire and left until it was charcoal-black and swollen. There were no eyes, no nose, no ears, no hair, no mouth, nothing except for this black charcoal mess sitting on my husband's shoulders. I was patting him on the only place I could see that wasn't burned. I knew that any moment I would faint; so I bent my head down toward the floor and kept patting him gently.

"Yes, honey, we're here."

The room was whirling now and I had to get away. I wanted to stay. I wanted to be strong, to stand by his side, to help him as he had often helped me in times of crises, but I could not make it.

"I'll be right back, Merrill," I said. "I am going to the hall for a moment."

I barely made it from the room before I collapsed. The doctor caught me as I fell. He, Wayne, and Chris all worked to revive me. Wayne knew of my history of heart problems, and the doctor could not get any pulse or blood-pressure signs. Then, as suddenly as I had fainted, I revived. For a moment all seemed normal. Then I pictured Merrill in my mind, lying on that bed, burned and bloody, and I fainted again.

This humiliating process went on for several minutes. Slowly I regained my composure. One thought made the difference. Merrill needed me. I hate to admit it, but during our first years of marriage I often secretly wondered if he needed me at all. He was so able and energetic and untiring. Now he was helpless and I was needed. This was no time for hysterical fainting spells.

"Wayne and Chris are here, honey," I said, returning to his

room and mustering up a halfway cheerful tone.

Immediately Merrill began to talk business. He was temporarily blind. He spoke through painful, swollen lips but he had written up five new orders for installations on his last trip. One of the orders in Redding, California, needed volume controls for speakers in cemetery trees, and Merrill leaned up on one elbow to explain thoroughly the installation problems.

I watched Wayne and Chris staring in disbelief as Merrill, blind, swollen, and still bleeding, gestured with enthusiasm and described the crash in detail. They didn't expect him to survive. They didn't expect to see him alive again, yet here he was on his deathbed—talking business follow-up letters, new ideas for National Music Service, and shouting, "Boy, did I hit hard." When Merrill had finished passing on to Wayne and Chris all the information and ideas he had stored in his mind, he settled back against the pillow exhausted.

A nurse moved us out into the hall. We took off the hospital gowns and headed into the cold evening air. Wayne and Chris insisted on feeding me one good meal before they returned to Spokane. I didn't want to eat. My stomach was still churning with what I had seen. Still, they ordered a hamburger steak for me. When the waitress brought the meat and set it before me, I burst out in tears again. It looked like Merrill's face.

There was a grim little motel about half a block from the hospital and they checked me in there and said good-by. They had their job to do now, and I had mine. But as they walked away I felt like yelling, "Don't leave me alone." Maybe other women are prepared to take charge. I was not. All my life my father and then my husband had made the major decisions, taken all the important steps. Now suddenly, without training, it was my turn. And I was scared. I couldn't even stay in that creepy little motel without feeling desperate and alone. Returning to the hospital, I made a bed out of hospital chairs and stayed right in Merrill's room.

* * * * *

VIRGINIA'S PRESENCE IN THAT room made a big difference for me. The first hours were filled with phone calls and reunions and excitement. Then the pain set in. People ask me how it feels to be so seriously burned. If you've ever been burned at all, just multiply that feeling all over your face, hands, and legs. Klamath Falls didn't have a burn ward or burn specialists, but they did what they could. They wrapped my hands and legs in gauze. They were afraid to wrap my face for fear of suffocation. They had never handled burns like these, but were smart enough to change the dressings on my hands two times a day. The leg dressings were not changed, and the gauze was absorbed by the scabs and pulled down into the burns. There are still gauze prints on my legs today.

They put a cast on one leg to keep it immobile. I couldn't understand why, because I hadn't broken any bones. Apparently blood clots were forming in my legs. They were using Dicumarol to thin my blood and prevent further clotting. I thought I was getting better, but the infection and the phlebitis signalled that I was getting worse.

The days and nights all blurred together. My eyes were swollen shut. I could only see shadows entering my room and departing again. Doctor shadows came with polite questions and gentle probings. Nurse shadows followed with needles and clean dressings and dextrose bottles for intravenous feedings. The noises in the hall seemed louder and more ominous as the shadows whispered to each other about my worsening condition. And through most of it, Virginia sat by my side. I would often awaken from a drugged sleep, call out to her, and fall asleep again.

3

Given the Choice—I Would Live

DURING THOSE LONG MISERABLE nights in the hospital I would watch my husband fighting to survive the shock and pain of those terrible burns. His face had swollen so badly that I couldn't see his eyes to know if he was awake or asleep. When I wasn't dozing fitfully, I would stare at him and pray. I didn't know what to pray for, so I repeated over and over, "Dear God, please help Merrill."

The second night, about two A.M., the hospital grew strangely silent. I sensed Merrill had awakened, and began patting him lightly on the shoulder. When he spoke that night it was as though I were in the darkness and only he could see. His words were clear. His mind was not befuddled. This was no dream, no drug-induced hallucination.

"Honey," he said, "I wish you could see what I can see right now."

The room was dark. His eyes were closed.

"What do you see?" I asked him.

"I see the bluest blue that I have ever seen in my life, and the greenest green. There is a hill and at the bottom of the hill there is a beautiful blue river. The river is lined with green trees, and above it all a blue sky."

For a moment he paused, as though staring at this incredibly beautiful scene and drinking it in. I quit patting him and gripped his shoulder lightly. I was afraid and yet strangely calm. He continued.

"There is a boat on the water," he whispered, "and a man in the boat."

27

Again he grew silent, concentrating, focusing on the boat and the man in the boat.

"Virginia, the man is Jesus, and He is motioning for me to get into the boat."

I felt a sob catch in my throat. This is it. I had heard about the mysterious moment of death and how it can be accompanied by a strange and beautiful vision. I was afraid Merrill was going to get into that boat on that beautiful river and leave me alone.

Merrill grew restless. I could feel his body tighten.

"What will you do, Merrill?"

"I don't know," he answered. "It is tearing me apart. I can go down the hill and get in the boat with Him or I can stay. It is so beautiful. There is a house on the other side of the river. I would like to go with Him, but I would also like to stay with you and the children. I don't know what to do."

That moment was incredibly real to both of us. God was giving Merrill the opportunity to choose between life or death, between the years of painful surgery and ugly scars or escape from all that. I knew how desperately I wanted him to stay with us; yet it had to be his decision.

"Merrill, it would be lovely to go with Jesus," I said, "but we need you here, too. Dan and Judie and Marlene need a dad. I need you. Hang on, because we want you as well. We all love you."

I felt the tears begin running down my cheeks. I wanted to hold him and keep him from getting into that boat. I wanted to fight off anyone or anything that would take him from me, but I had to let him go. I had been praying that God would take care of Merrill. Now it was time for me to believe that God was able to do just that.

"We want you to stay with us, honey, but do what you feel you must do."

*   *   *   *   *

I KNEW WHAT I WOULD DO. I would live. I had been given the choice and I would live. The room was dark again. That beautiful pastoral scene faded as quickly as it had appeared. The lush green meadow, the tree-covered hill, the crystal-blue river, and the man beckoning to me from the boat in the river all disappeared.

The next morning I heard the doctor telling Virginia that I had been on the threshold of death. He had left me the evening before wondering if I would make it through the night. Now that crisis was over. Through that vision I had been offered a choice. My decision was now made. I believe that God knew about the long years of suffering ahead and that night gave me the choice to accept or reject that suffering.

My reveries were interrupted when a new morning nurse placed another bottle of dextrose on the long metal hanger and then nervously jammed the feed needle back into my arm, trying to find a healthy vein.

"Sorry," she mumbled and quickly left the room.

Just outside the door she stopped and began chatting with an orderly. The door was open enough for me to hear their whispered conversation.

"Have you seen that horrible-looking creature in there?" she said. "I can hardly touch him."

They walked away whispering. I could hear their footsteps disappearing down the long hospital corridor. A doctor was being paged. A cart rattled by outside. Nothing had changed, yet my spirit sagged.

Have you seen that horrible-looking creature?

I knew how bad I felt, but I had never really seen how bad I looked. Apparently Virginia suspected this would happen one day and had removed the mirror from the room. Now she was next door at a restaurant having coffee. I was alone and had to see for myself. I forced open one eye with my bandaged fingers and tried to find a reflective surface. On my nightstand a shiny

chrome tray served as a makeshift mirror. I leaned down awk-
wardly over that tray. The face staring back at me out of that
fun-house mirror was not mine. What I saw was horrible. I *was*
ugly. I was a horrible-looking creature, and I knew in that moment that I would never look the same again. I was a singer and
a salesman. My life depended on making a good impression on
people, and even a nurse trained for tragedy could not bear to
look at me. I slumped back on the bed just as Virginia entered
the room again. She could tell that something was wrong.

"What's the matter, honey?" she asked.

I did not want to admit my feelings. I was embarrassed and
angry and shocked.

"Nothing is wrong," I answered, turning away.

"Well, something is wrong," she gently coaxed me. "What
happened while I was gone?"

Finally I blurted out, "How can you stand by me when I am
such a horrible-looking creature?"

She paused for one long, thoughtful moment, "Merrill, I love
you for what is inside you, not for what is outside."

I needed that. She did not pretend. She did not deny. I had an
ugly, burned face, but I was not an ugly person. My face was
gone, but I was still there inside the black burned shell that
remained. I had not changed, and Virginia still loved me. There
were rough, embarrassing times ahead when others would not be
so gracious in their shock and surprise at seeing me. The hospital
hired a special night nurse with thirteen years of experience to
change my dressings and monitor my vital signs. She entered my
room the first time, took one look at me and walked out past the
supervisor who had just hired her—without even saying good-by.

I was a terrible sight. There are no pictures of those first
horrible weeks at Klamath Falls, no way to illustrate how bad I
looked. My head was swollen larger than a basketball. The ears,
nose, eyebrows—in fact, most of the bumps and folds we call a
face—were burned off. The flesh scabbed over. The scabs would

break and leave my face covered with bloody, oozing pus and then scab over again. My hands were like ugly blood-red claws. Yet Virginia never turned away, and her words, "I love you for what is inside you, not for what is outside," got me through the shock and embarrassment I felt as others looked at the surface —and turned away.

It was not all grim, even during those first horrible days near death. Only a day before the accident I had been sitting in the office of C.J. Ward, a funeral director in Klamath Falls. While he finished up some telephone business, I thumbed through a pile of funeral directors' cards which I carry in my pocket for reference. Our company provides music to funeral homes, and these directors are my primary customers. As Mr. Ward hung up the phone he noticed me thumbing through the cards.

"Merrill, why in the world do you carry all those old business cards?" he asked.

"They're funeral directors' cards," I answered, "and the one I fall closest to can take care of me." He laughed and handed me his card. "Who knows," he teased, "maybe I'll get lucky."

A week after my accident the receptionist in the hospital would have been horrified to see funeral director Ward sneaking past her checkpoint after visiting hours, card in hand. Silently he slipped into my room, put the card on my table, and whispered, "Merrill, you awake?"

"C.J., how did you get in here?" I asked, recognizing his voice.

"Well, you fell nearest me, so I've come to take care of you," he answered. For a moment there was silence, then we both began to laugh.

* * * * *

IT WAS NOT EASY for me to laugh during those first eleven days. Usually when Merrill gets under pressure, instead of yelling or getting moody, he gets the giggles and acts crazy. I just bottle up my emotions and hold back the tears. After that first fainting spell in the hospital corridor, I did not allow myself to cry again. It was my time to be strong, I reasoned. Merrill needs me to be his strength. No more fainting spells, no more tears. But now and then when I would visit that damp, grim motel room to change my clothes and take a bath, I would sit staring into the mirror and want to cry.

"You're just feeling sorry for yourself," I muttered. "Merrill's doing the suffering and you want to cry. Shame on you."

"But I am suffering, too," I argued to myself, "and nobody understands my suffering."

"Suffering? You have it made. You aren't burned. You haven't lost your looks."

"Maybe not," I answered that voice inside me, "but I am suffering nevertheless. I have lost a husband. At least for this moment he is helpless and for the first time in my life I am in charge. And I'm not ready for it." No one prepared me to make decisions. My father made the decisions in my childhood. My husband took his place and had been making the decisions ever since. Even in the small things, the men in my life had made all the choices.

"Where shall we go for dinner, Virginia?"

"Anywhere you like, dear."

It became a ritual and I rarely if ever said what I wanted to do or made any decisions on my own. I suppose I was an old-fashioned woman that way. I was married on my nineteenth birthday. We had our first baby when I was still nineteen. I went to college only one year and then dropped out to have our family. I just took it for granted that home was my place. I never questioned it. Merrill went out into the world. I stayed home to raise the children. My place was in the kitchen baking cookies, in the bathroom scrubbing tiles, or in their bedrooms hearing the children's heartaches, wrapping skinned knees, and talking about schools and dates and daydreams. My life was wrapped up in my husband, my children, and my home. I was happy to have Merrill do all the rest.

Now I had to take over. I had to decide about doctors and operations. I needed to find a plastic surgeon and a burn ward. I had to pay the bills and keep the family together. I even had to find and hire an air ambulance for the long trip home.

All these choices were foreign to me. I was frightened, like a lost child who did not know what corner to turn to find her way home again. Merrill was my life. And as he lay near death in that hospital bed I was not sure how long "my life" was going to be.

He received hundreds of letters and telegrams and phone calls during those first days. I received none. At first I felt abandoned and unimportant. Of course, running myself down had always been my way of responding to life. I was not a fantastic housekeeper. I was not a fantastic wife. I even felt guilty because I had two premature children and cheated them on their full nine-month terms. In my mind I had been a failure and had no real purpose in life.

Now suddenly all that was changing. Whether I liked it or not, I was in control of both our lives. Merrill was hurt. Merrill needed me. As I sat in that little motel room staring down at the timid, unprepared, inadequate, helpless little woman in the mirror, I knew that at last I had found my work. I only wished I had prepared for it along the way.

Those first nights in Klamath Falls were particularly frightening because the doctor confided in me about Merrill's condition. The internal bleeding and the phlebitis were weakening him, and they could not treat these conditions adequately in Klamath. Yet he could not be moved until his face scabbed over, or infection would set in and kill him. It was a real predicament—to know that he couldn't stay and he couldn't be moved—to know that he might be dying and if he lived he would be terribly scarred. This was the first time in our marriage that I knew something he could not know. It was a tragic secret I had to bear alone. I was scared to death to be there by myself in that hospital at night because I thought any minute I would really be alone. Still I had to take charge, to make decisions, and to make them on my own.

After eleven days of awful waiting and hoping and praying, Merrill's face scabbed over adequately for the emergency flight to Spokane. Now the decision was mine. I had to sign the release. I had to make arrangements for the air ambulance. I had to contact burn specialists in Spokane and find a plastic surgeon. I had to get Merrill admitted to the hospital and find an ambulance to meet us at the airport. It was all a bit overwhelming at first, but I began to feel more and more confident after each new decision. I was learning to be responsible. I had no choice. Merrill couldn't make all the decisions now, and it was exciting to see myself beginning to change. The woman I was eleven days before— fainting in the hospital corridor and overwhelmed by the loneliness, the helplessness and the terror of it all—was becoming a new woman, a grown-up, a person. And though my knees still knocked from time to time, and though some of my decisions would be wrong, I was alive. I had found a new purpose. I hated for him to suffer, to be helpless and immobile, but I was beginning to discover that I, too, had strength. The hope began to dawn in me that I could be a strong and decisive human being.

* * * * *

I THOUGHT THE REASON Virginia was transferring me to Spokane was that I was getting better. The real reason was that I was getting worse—from the phlebitis condition in my legs. The doctor had been using a blood thinner to keep the clots from forming, but the blood-thinning process was causing me serious internal bleeding. There was no specialist in Klamath Falls who could take care of me then—so at last we were given the go-ahead to fly home.

Virginia hired an air ambulance. When we pulled up on the airstrip beside that bright red 310 Cessna, I wanted to fly again, at least to sit up front with the pilot, but the doctor wouldn't let me. In fact, the doctor flew with us in case I needed a shot, and

Virginia sat in front with the pilot. Everyone thought I would be afraid to go up in a plane again. I forced my eyes open from time to time on that flight and even pointed out directions along the way. As we neared the Spokane field, the pilot couldn't remember the radio frequency; so I gave him the frequency to the tower. It felt great to be flying again, even as a backseat pilot.

As we taxied up to the waiting ambulance I jumped out of the airplane and walked over to the rolling stretcher they had prepared. I had no idea that I was in danger of blood clots and just ignored the doctor's warning to prevent any movement in the leg at all.

As I lay down on the stretcher, the sheets blew off. For a moment I lay on that stretcher with all my burns exposed. At that moment my father walked around the ambulance from where he had been waiting to greet me. He took one look at me and began to cry. He never really recovered from that first painful look. Others who knew me before I lost my face reacted with pity and sorrow at that first sight. It is too bad that none of us could understand then how God would use this accident and the years of painful surgery that lay ahead to bring new insight, new hope, and healing to all our lives.

4

I Would Never Leave Him

A YOUNG AMBULANCE ATTENDANT hurried to Merrill's side and covered his burns with a sterile sheet. Quickly he and the driver lifted my husband into the ambulance and secured the rolling cart in place. From where I stood watching, the sheet-covered body looked like a corpse. As they slammed the doors and rushed by me to start the ambulance and drive away, I cried out.

"He's my husband. I want to go with him."

The attendant turned back and helped me in beside Merrill. I fastened the seat belt just as the ambulance turned onto the street near the airport and sped towards the Deaconess Hospital in Spokane.

The siren screamed out the agony I felt riding beside my husband that day. How many times we had driven those same streets together on the way to a family dinner, to the airport, or just for a Sunday afternoon ride around town. Spokane is a beautiful city. The Spokane River flows through the heart of the business district down a series of natural falls, deep pools, and crystal rapids. But that day nothing seemed familiar. Nothing seemed beautiful. We passed people in the streets, browsing through the shops, eating at restaurants, or just chatting with passing friends. They did not even look up as we sped by. I suppose that is the way I would have responded before Merrill's crash. Now when an ambulance goes by or a siren sounds I always pause to pray, "God be with them, whoever they are!"

We turned onto Fourth Street and into the emergency receiving area of the hospital. Several orderlies hurried up to assist the attendants. Hands reached out and took my husband from the ambulance. Struggling with the seat belt, I felt desperate as though they were taking him from me again. Hospital personnel were everywhere. Orderlies transferred Merrill to a guerny cart. Fresh sterile sheets were draped over him. A nurse attached a new plasma bottle to his arm. Again they were wheeling him away. They had cleared the hall of all traffic to help prevent the chance of infection. Patients who saw Merrill pass turned away in shock and surprise. I felt like I was in a nightmare. My legs were heavy. I could not keep up with all those uniformed men and women determined to take my husband from me. Finally I slumped into a chair in the waiting room.

I felt like crying. My eyes filled with tears. I began to feel faint, when suddenly I remembered that woman in Klamath Falls, unconscious in the hospital corridor. I must not succumb to self-pity or to fear again. I must not panic. This was the second step on my road to becoming a person. And though the environment had changed, and though the problems that lay ahead were looming large, I must face them.

Besides, I was not alone. All my life I had lived with people who believed in God. I had sung their hymns. I had prayed their prayers. I had quoted their verses. Now it was time for me to quit parroting others' religious experiences. It was time to test my own faith. If there was a God and if that God really helps people in times of tragedy and fear, then that same God could help me.

As I sat there in that hospital waiting room, surrounded by strangers and feeling terribly alone, I thought of a Bible verse learned years before in Sunday School, "I can do all things through Christ who strengthens me" (*see* Philippians 4:13). I whispered it over and over to myself. *I can do all things through Christ who strengthens me.* He had been with me in Klamath Falls during those past eleven horrible days. Now He would be with me again in Spokane. It was amazing how that one line from the Bible jogged my memory and started hope flowing in me again.

"Mrs. Womach, please come to the hospital admissions office."

I heard my name called through the hospital paging system and hurried to the office. There were endless forms to be filled out and credit checks to be made. There were references to be noted and phone numbers to recall.

At first my hand trembled slightly. I could not remember my own address or telephone number. I sat staring down at that pile of unfriendly papers. Merrill had always done this kind of thing for me. I didn't even know my Social Security number or our hospitalization plan. What would I do? Then those words came to me again—*I can do all things through Christ who strengthens me.* My trembling stopped. I remembered my phone number, and somehow miraculously got through the rest of those long, complicated forms.

*   *   *   *   *

WHILE VIRGINIA WAS STRUGGLING to complete the hospital admission process, I was being wheeled into my room on the fifth floor. My eyes were still swollen shut but I used a bandaged hand to force one eye open. There were yellow tiles on the floors and walls. Green curtains hung from the windows. The room was bright and cheery.

Just then a nurse entered the room and plugged in the telephone I had ordered upon arrival. I was ready to begin doing business again. Soon life would be back to normal and my family and I would be reunited in our home. In my excitement at being in Spokane, and still under the influence of a strong dose of painkiller, I really thought the nightmare had ended. In fact, it had just begun.

Across from my bed, on the wall above a dressing table, hung a mirror. I sat up slowly, remembering the doctor's warning about using my legs, and strained to see my reflection in the mirror. I could not believe what I saw staring back at me from the wall that day.

My face was charcoal-black. My nose was gone. Little stumps of burned flesh hung where my ears had been. I was forcing my left eye open, but my right eye was missing, buried somewhere under a mass of swollen, oozing tissue. There were no eyelids or eyebrows. My hair had been singed away and my head was gigantic, like a huge Halloween pumpkin. I looked exactly like a marshmallow that had been dropped into a campfire, or a monster oozing up out of a swamp in a Japanese horror film. My normally white skin was charred, wrinkled, and still bleeding. My hands were clawlike, black, and ugly.

For a moment I stared at the thing in the mirror. As I fell back onto the pillows it was very plain that the family reunion was not soon to be. I knew then this bright, cheery little room would be my home for many months, but I still felt at peace. There was some shock at seeing how badly I had been burned. There was also some fear in not knowing if at any moment a blood clot might break free and kill me. But there was an even greater sense of peace in knowing that God was with me and would get me through whatever pain or problem lay ahead.

"Hello, Merrill."

A new voice interrupted the silence. I reached up to force my eye open again.

"Don't do that, friend."

Whoever was speaking to me was obviously in charge.

"Hello, Doctor," I answered, lowering my arm back into place. "How soon are you going to have me out of here?"

The doctor laughed quietly.

"As soon as we can," he replied. "I can't have you around too long depressing the other patients with those burns of yours."

"Are they as bad as they look?" I asked.

"Merrill," he answered, "a plastic surgeon could go a lifetime and not see anyone as badly burned as you are, but we have all kinds of new equipment and techniques to heal and rebuild your face and I can't wait to get started."

Saying that, he leaned over me and began to probe gently, determining what damage had been done, deciding what treatment would be followed. I liked his honesty and felt hope coming from him. He asked questions about the crash, about the flames, about the snow, about the ride to Klamath Falls and the hospital there. He even asked if I took aspirins for a headache. Then, as suddenly as he had appeared, he was gone.

Moments later nurses swarmed in and began following his instructions. The gauze that had not been absorbed into my leg burns was removed inch by inch with forceps and scissors. Bottles containing nutrients were hung, and needles were poked into my veins and taped snugly into place. The nurses talked quietly, worked quickly and efficiently. But it was obvious that they thought I was unconscious. I had not spoken and my eyes were buried beneath the burnt flesh. Although my face was too swollen to speak normally, I used my old ventriloquist skills to greet them.

"Hi, girls," I said, and at least three nurses gasped in chorus. "Mr. Womach, we thought you were sleeping."

"How can I," I replied, "when you girls insist on smoking cigars while you are working on me!"

The nurses laughed. There was a strong smell of cigar smoke in the room and I had noticed it about the time they arrived.

"You can always tell when Dr. Hamacher is on call," one explained. "He is a great plastic surgeon and he spends so much time with patients and their families that he has to smoke on the run."

"He leaves his cigar just outside a patient's room," another nurse interrupted, "then picks it up when he leaves again."

"That way," laughed the third nurse, "by the time any smell gets inside the room he's gone and we get the blame."

It was easy to feel how those nurses admired Dr. Hamacher by the affectionate way they discussed his one bad habit. I never liked cigar smoke before my accident, but during those long days in the hospital, that smell became a helpful warning that my surgeon was in the area checking up on me, and a symbol of his constant, caring presence.

*   *   *   *   *

AFTER FINISHING THE ADMISSION forms, I waited to meet the plastic surgeon who would attend Merrill during the years of treatment that lay ahead. The waiting room was almost empty when he entered. He wore a long green surgical gown. A mask dangled around his neck. He stood at the door looking down at me for the longest time before he spoke. I felt for a moment as if I were the patient, that I was about to be operated on. Then he smiled and sat down beside me.

"Mrs. Womach," he began, "I don't know you. I don't know your husband. I don't know how much you love each other or how healthy your marriage is. But I do know one thing. If you are thinking of leaving him now because he is so badly burned and can never look the same again, you had better tell me."

I was stunned. It wasn't the opening line I had expected. Yet he sat looking at me, totally serious and awaiting my reply.

"Leave him?" I finally blurted out. "That's the furthest thing from my mind. I love him whatever he looks like and I would never leave him."

"Good," he answered. "You can visit your husband now. Come to my office this afternoon around three o'clock and we'll talk." With that he was gone.

Later that day he explained to me why he asked that strange question about our marriage. Apparently the husbands or wives of patients with accidental or surgical deformities often recoil at their partner's mishap. It sometimes happens that one who has had a breast removed or a face deformed or even a scar resulting from an operation or accident loses his loved one in the process. Out of shock or embarrassment or disappointment, the one needed most to comfort and sustain the victim runs from the scene, leaving the patient alone and in another kind of shock. The shock that comes from being abandoned can seriously hamper the patient's treatment and even kill him. Dr. Hamacher wanted to know at the outset if I was considering leaving Merrill, because that problem, too, must be figured into his total treatment strategy.

Many times I walked down that hospital corridor past all those patients alone in their rooms and wondered if they had been abandoned by their loved ones. I remembered others in my life who had been in this same hospital, dying from cancer or suffering through long, painful illnesses. I had sent a card or made one quick courtesy call, but in fact I had abandoned them. I had used my busy schedule, my growing family, or my obligations at church as excuses not to visit, when in fact I was embarrassed. I didn't know what to say. So I said nothing. I didn't know what to do. So I disappeared. Dr. Hamacher taught me that the ones we love and their reactions and responses to us in times of crises are as important a part of our healing as the medicine prescribed.

Merrill was on the fifth floor, and after the elevator ride, the quick instructions from the nurses at the nursing station, and the long walk to his room, I stood at the door looking down at my husband. He would have excellent surgeons, he would have trained, competent nurses, he would have the best in facilities and in care, but that was not enough. He would have me, too— loving, hoping, caring, and praying at every step along the way.

I don't like hospitals. I hate to be around suffering. I find it difficult to make small talk day after day and to be cheerful when constantly sitting and waiting and suffering through hours of painful boredom. There are times I would have rather been the patient than the wife or the husband who waits. No one prepares us to be a victim's friend. No one helps us know how to wait. Yet I am now convinced that our role is equally important to the doctor or the nurse directly involved in the treatment of those we love.

"Hi, Merrill, I'm back."

"Virginia, I love you."

5

His Faith Was Contagious

ONE NIGHT IN SPOKANE I awakened from a drug-induced sleep. My body ached. The burns throbbed painfully. I felt terribly weak. Two men were quietly discussing my condition. Because I recognized Dr. Hamacher's voice I was afraid to force open one eye to identify the other doctor. It was easy to sense their tension. Something had gone wrong. I could feel the pain, but was not sure why I was hurting so.

"What's the matter, Dr. Hamacher?" I asked.

Their voices stopped. Hamacher moved over to my side.

"Sorry we wakened you, Merrill, but your internal hemorrhaging has gotten worse. Your blood pressure is decreasing and you've thrown a little plugger or blood clot."

"So what does that mean?" I asked.

"It means that my friend here will have to tie off a vein in your leg to keep another clot from going to your lungs and causing real damage."

"But what about the plastic surgery?" I asked. "When can you get started on my new face?"

"That will have to wait," said the second voice, "until the venacavaligation helps prevent further embolisms and stabilizes the phlebitis condition."

With that the other doctor walked from the room.

I was wondering to myself why so many doctors speak Latin to patients dying in English, when Hamacher leaned down and whispered, "Don't worry, Merrill. He's a great surgeon even if he can't speak English. Anyway, I'll be along to translate." He laughed, patted me on the shoulder and started to walk from the room.

"By the way, he is a very serious fellow in surgery. Try to cheer him up a bit, won't you?"

Then he was gone. Immediately Virginia was by my side. She did not say much during those times of crises, but she was always there and it made such a difference.

* * * * *

WHAT COULD I SAY? I didn't know then what a venacavaligation meant. I'm still not sure how veins are tied off, how blood is thinned, or how clots are thrown. Merrill always wanted to know what was going to happen. I was glad just to learn that it was over and that he was still alive.

Earlier in the day Merrill had complained of chest pains. I hurried to the pay phone in the waiting room and called Dr. Hamacher. Marlene and Judie both had music lessons scheduled for that afternoon so I reassured Merrill that Hamacher was on his way and that I would return immediately after delivering our daughters to their respective classes. However, I hardly got inside our front door before the hospital called and urged my immediate return. Merrill needed emergency surgery. Blood clots were massing dangerously near his heart.

In numb shock I raced to the car and drove back towards Deaconess Hospital. In my haste I forgot my purse in the living room and only remembered it as I pulled into the toll booth on the Maple Street Bridge. Frantically I yelled to the attendant.

"I've forgotten my purse. I'll pay twice next time! Merrill's in emergency. . . ." The young man knew me well, having read about Merrill's crash and seeing me cross the bridge back and forth between the hospital as many as ten times a day.

"Go on, Mrs. Womach. It's 'on the house.'"

I waved gratefully just as my side-view mirror caught the

change box and sent it crashing to the ground. The attendant scrambled after the falling coins and waved me on. "Don't worry about it," he yelled. I could see him in the rearview mirror, shaking his head and thinking awful thoughts about women drivers.

The hospital parking lot was full, so I double-parked, ran through the lobby, and got off the elevator just as the orderly wheeled Merrill away towards surgery. I never got used to that feeling of being parted even temporarily. I know it is silly, but every time someone wheeled him away I felt like running after them yelling, "I love you, Merrill. Don't die." Instead, I walked slowly to the surgical waiting room or to the coffee shop to sit and to wait. I had faith that God would take care of Merrill, and at the same time I wondered if Merrill would die. Isn't that what faith is—being confident and yet wondering? Sometimes religious writers and speakers make me feel guilty for those moments of fear or doubt. Now, looking back, I am convinced that faith is not the absence of fear or doubt, but the force that gets you safely through those long, dark waiting-room hours.

Waiting rooms are awful places. Clocks lose time there! The magazines are old and already read. The coffee gets cold and tastes bitter. The television set has some old movie or game show playing that I never quite figure out. Even the commercials don't make sense. And every time a voice pages doctors to surgery or when nurses wheel elaborate equipment rapidly down the hall, I am convinced that whatever the emergency, Merrill is probably in the middle of it.

That first surgery was no exception. I paced and sat. I prayed and worried. I bought coffee and let it get cold. I reread ancient versions of the *National Geographic* and recalled Scripture verses. Then I paced and sat some more.

Finally, Dr. Hamacher entered the room, smiling broadly.

"Virginia, you should have been there."

I started to ask him why I should have been there, but he interrupted me.

"It was one of the most incredible things I have ever seen. Merrill was lying on the operating table. We had given him a local anesthetic and my serious surgeon friend was beginning his work. Suddenly Merrill began to sing. You should have seen him lying there badly burned and bleeding, and the surgeon going through his stomach to tie off his veins, with Merrill singing old gospel songs at the top of his lungs."

"How is he, Dr. Hamacher?"

"He's great, Virginia; I've never heard a better singer."

"No," I said, "How was the vena-cava-whatever? How is he doing?"

"Oh, he's fine, but my serious doctor friend will never be the same. He actually smiled during one of those gospel songs."

Merrill knew that one little embolism thrown into his lungs or one little blood clot to the brain could have meant instant death, and yet he sang. It became a tradition in that hospital over the next twelve years. Whenever Merrill came for surgery, nurses gathered around in hopes he would sing those gospel songs again.

*   *   *   *   *

I WANTED TO SING! I believe that God is at work in every moment of our lives. If we live or die—if one has a face burned off or is rescued from the flames without a trace of smoke—God is there, loving and caring for us. I quit trying to figure out why He does some things and why He seems unwilling to do others. For me the *why* questions lead nowhere. It is enough for me to know that God is at work in my life. Even when the pain comes, God is there, and that is why I sing. He is at work in my life for good even when it seems bad to me. Believing that God is not there or that He does not care leads only to loneliness and despair. I would rather sing.

During this crisis there were many signs of God's presence in our lives. I am a shirt-sleeve pilot. At the time of my accident I had flown 1,500 hours in all kinds of airplanes. Since the accident

I have accumulated another 4,100 flying hours in everything from Piper Cubs to Saberliner jets, and not one time in all of this flying have I ever flown an airplane with my coat on. I feel tied up in a cockpit when I am wearing a coat. So, as a matter of habit, I remove my jacket before entering the plane.

I can recall only one exception to this rule in all my years of flying. That was the day I crashed at Beaver Marsh. That morning I took off with my coat on. It was not because it was cold. In fact, I had flown the day before in the middle of a snowstorm in my shirt-sleeves. My airplane had a heavy-duty Southwind gas heater that even in its lowest notch got so hot that I felt uncomfortable in the cockpit. But somehow that day I wore my coat. If I had not, I would not have survived.

When I crashed into the trees and the airplane exploded, everything burned. My face burned, as did my hair and my hands. My trousers were made of woolen material and they burned away completely, leaving bad scars on my legs. Even the shoes that I was wearing were burned, and I still have scars on the tops and bottoms of my feet. Underneath my jacket that day was a nylon wash-and-wear shirt. Imagine how that shirt would have burned if my jacket had not been made of some synthetic material that was transformed into an asbestoslike covering by the intense flames. The doctor in Klamath Falls had to cut the jacket away; it became so hard in the fire.

In the plastic surgery that lay ahead, all the skin used to rebuild my face and hands came from areas protected by that flame-hardened jacket. My forehead and my temple came from the right side of my body. The chin and cheeks came from across the center of my stomach. My neck came from my lower stomach, and my nose and eyelids came from the upper parts of my arms. The skin of my right hand came from the right side of my body, and the skin of my left hand came from the left side. No one yet has been able to explain to me how that synthetic jacket turned hard and protected me. I believe it was all a part of God's incredible plan, and that wearing my jacket that day was nothing short of a miracle.

There are other examples I could cite. The doctors were amazed by my singing, not just because I sang during surgery but that I could sing at all. To crash in flames and not to have burned or bruised those delicate vocal folds that produce song is a miracle. To struggle at escaping from the burning plane and not singe my lungs is another miracle. Apparently, as the plane began to crash, I tucked my neck down into my chest and raised my arms just long enough to trap a layer of protective air that shielded my lungs and vocal cords from the incredible heat. I believe this, too, was an act of God, and a definite part of His plan for me.

* * * * *

EVEN DURING THOSE FIRST days in Spokane when Merrill had blood clots, serious hemorrhaging, open, bleeding burns, and intense, relentless pain, it seemed easy for me to trust God. Merrill was almost always cheerful and confident. He did not spend a lot of time thinking about his tragedy. He never asked why. He just believed. For others it was not so easy.

The third day in Spokane, Merrill learned that a dear clergyman friend was in the hospital being treated for a sinus infection and exhaustion. Merrill had been wheeled to X-ray and insisted on seeing his friend on the return trip. Several months later the clergyman reported to his entire congregation what happened during Merrill's surprise visit.

"There I was," the clergyman told his congregation, "feeling so sorry for myself, lying in that hospital room, suffering only from a bad case of discouragement, when Merrill was wheeled into my room. I didn't even recognize him. His face was gone and he was wrapped in bandages.

" 'Hey, brother, I hope you're feeling better,' he called out, and I immediately recognized Merrill's voice. I had heard he had been burned, but the shock of seeing how badly burned he really was made me feel faint. There he was, his face burned black. He was blind. His lips were gone and his head swollen so badly he looked inhuman; yet he sat in my room encouraging me, wishing me well. Hospital personnel were not sure that Merrill could survive the surgery ahead. They did not know if he would live or die, and as the orderly wheeled him out of my room again, Merrill shouted back over his shoulder, 'Have a good day!' "

As he stood before his congregation telling of Merrill's visit to his room, tears streamed down his face. "I was the man of faith, and I was only suffering from exhaustion, yet seeing his terrible burns gave me a relapse. I was supposed to leave the hospital that day, yet I went into shock after seeing Merrill's condition and had to stay several more days to recuperate."

This clergyman's reaction to Merrill's burns was not unusual. Everyone who visited him during those first days in Spokane went away feeling shocked by the seriousness of his condition and amazed at his faith in the face of suffering. The fourth night in the hospital, I sat in his room watching him sleep. The face I had known and loved was gone. The lips that I had kissed so many times had been charred black by the flames. The thick wavy hair was burned away. I could not recognize the man I married. Yet I knew it was still Merrill lying on that bed—from the way he refused to give in to the pain he felt or to the horror that lay ahead.

From his childhood he had been one who refused to quit or to give up in face of a struggle. His parents told me that as a young teenager Merrill tried out for the track team but was too small and too slightly built for the field events. Merrill wanted to pole-vault, but the coach rejected him first time around. To be considered for that event, the young athletes had to vault nine feet or more. Merrill sat in the bleachers that day watching the new team learn to pole-vault. At the end of the day he had listened carefully to the vaulters' questions and to the coach's replies. He followed the coach to the office and asked to borrow one of the old worn vaulting poles. Finally, under pressure, the coach gave in to the young boy's request and Merrill lugged that long pole to his home across town.

During the next few weeks, everyone in the neighborhood saw a strange sight. Merrill was only five feet four inches tall and weighed only ninety-eight pounds. When he first tried to lift and balance that long springy pole, he looked awkward and off-balance. He would pick it up and try to run with it, but the front end would catch in the weeds as he ran, and toss him to the ground. Neighbors laughed and pointed as Merrill ran up and down the vacant lot carrying that ridiculous old taped-together pole. Time and time again he would drop the pole, walk away from it, and then quickly turn as if on cue and run back to the pole to pick it up. He was getting the feel. He was discovering the place of perfect balance.

He walked the pole around the neighborhood like others walked their dogs. He tried to vault over fences and ended up dangling from the wire mesh or slammed breathless against the wooden fencing. Still he tried. In Merrill's mind he was wearing his silk track suit and breaking school records before cheering schoolmates.

Little by little he got the feel of it. The neighbors quit laughing and began cheering him on. Little Merrill flew over fences, landing with a thud in backyards, bruised and shaken. He would run and jump until there wasn't a fence in Spokane he couldn't somehow get over.

The next year at the beginning of track season, Merrill was first in line. The coach rejected him again, but Merrill, undaunted, walked over to the vaulting area. Wearing his school clothes and heavy shoes, he picked up his pole and, balancing it as carefully as any Olympic champion, he ran and vaulted the nine-foot minimum with room to spare. The team cheered, the coach signed him up, and Merrill walked home smiling. Later that year Merrill tied for the city championship in pole-vaulting.

The perseverance that awed all of us who saw Merrill during his first years of suffering was not accidental. God was preparing him as a child to face hardship and not be conquered by it. By the time of the crash God had equipped my husband with strength and courage. I was not so well prepared. This was my first step in growing spiritual muscles. This was my pole-vault experience. Yet already I felt my strength growing. His faith was contagious and it spread to me. During the next few years I found myself able to do things that I never dreamed I could do.

6

Time to Cry

As I LAY IN THE HOSPITAL bed those first weeks in Spokane, I was grateful to be alive. More than seventy thousand people a year die in fires in this country before they can be hospitalized. I had miraculously escaped the flaming wreckage. I had been rescued from the snowbound woods of Oregon. I had received adequate emergency treatment in Klamath Falls and now I was a patient in a modern hospital with a great plastic surgeon. I was home, close to family and friends, and I was alive.

Still, there were times of depression. The phlebitis complication was slowing down the treatment of the burns. I lay there wanting desperately for Dr. Hamacher to begin the long process of grafting and rebuilding my face and hands. I had hopes then that plastic surgery could restore me to my normal appearance. I had heard of film stars and celebrities who had plastic surgery that made them look even better than when they started. My mind was filled with old myths about plastic surgery. I had no idea of the painfully slow and imperfect process that lay ahead.

At first we had to wait for granules of fresh, whole skin to grow in the burned areas. The dead skin had to be removed. The scabs being formed had to be picked off each day until the healed area could accept skin grafts removed from other parts of my body.

The nurses used to hesitate outside my room and take several deep breaths before entering. They needed that moment to steel themselves for the awful task of removing my dead tissue and the scabs forming over it. Even the most experienced registered nurse found the process difficult.

"Good morning, Mr. Womach." They tried to muster a cheerful tone, but I knew what was going on in their minds.

"We've come to do it again," they said.

I would groan playfully and protest, but it had to be done. Two hours a day the nurses would pull off the growing scabs with forceps. The nurses often shook so badly that they would accidentally stick me with their forceps and really hurt me in the process. Virginia finally asked to do it herself. The nurses were only too happy to be relieved from this unpleasant task.

Every day Virginia would prepare the dressings and the sterile forceps. Then a nurse would administer the strongest possible painkiller. As the shot took hold, Virginia would begin pulling off my skin. She tried to make a game of it.

"Oh, boy, Merrill, just got a big one. That's a record scab. Here's another."

It hurt like fury. Virginia would work as quickly as possible to get it finished. Three times a day she tugged and pulled the scabs away. Burned skin heals from the outside in, and the forming scabs would create problems for the grafting process. The scabs would get thick; sometimes half an inch or even an inch would form. We could not let them build up. This scar tissue had to be removed. Three times every day Virginia had to pull off my skin. As the forceps tore away the scabs, the new wound would bleed and have to be cleaned. Many times a day the sheets and pillowcases would be soaked in blood.

My hands needed similar treatment every day from the first. Virginia would put on her cap, gown, and rubber gloves. Then she would gently unwrap the gauze and dressings from my hands and soak them in a container that looked like a milk bucket. She moved them gently in the solution for fifteen or twenty minutes. After they had soaked, she would take my hands from the pan and with her own hands run down each of my individual fingers, wiping away the slimy dead skin that was forming there. It reminded me of milking a cow. If she hadn't done this, my hands would have grown together in webs like a duck's foot. The skin on my hands had been burned completely away. Virginia would wipe off each finger, apply ointment, and rewrap each finger in gauze. When she was finished my hands looked like large round mittens. This process went on two or three times each day.

The phlebitis condition in my leg had to be treated, too. The doctor provided a large heating pad with elements running through it filled with circulating hot water. Virginia would wrap my leg and this would make the blood flow more easily. They could not move my leg for fear of breaking loose the blood clots. So every hour Virginia would gently raise the leg onto a pillow or two and apply this heated water treatment. The operation had solved the problem of blood clots to my heart, because the two main veins that lead to the heart were tied off surgically. Yet the hot-water treatment was still necessary, sometimes day and night.

With burns there is another irritating problem. The burns smell sickeningly sweet. It is burnt flesh, after all, and the oozing pus has an odor of its own. The body is trying to slough off the dead tissue and heal the burns. Fortunately, Virginia didn't seem bothered by the burns or their treatment. She was incredibly tough through all of this.

She usually slept at home with the children. In the morning she would prepare the children's breakfast, get them off to school, then rush to the hospital to pull off scabs or soak and clean my hands. All day long she worked at making me comfortable. In the evenings she would prepare the children's meal and get them ready for bed. A neighbor helped watch the children in the evenings while Virginia bathed, changed, and rushed back to the hospital for my evening treatments. She removed my bloody sheets. She laughed and joked and prayed with me. She was strong and able and untiring. She seldom if ever complained.

*   *   *   *   *

I STAYED WITH MERRILL day and night those first weeks in Spokane. A wonderful neighbor helped with the children. I sometimes bathed and slept right in the hospital room. Those days were very difficult for me. I was needed, and yet I had no stomach for tearing scabs away or cleaning slimy fingers. It had to be done and it had to be done correctly. Merrill's life was at stake and some of the nurses had less stomach than I to get that close to those bleeding, oozing burns. So I did it.

I didn't complain and I didn't cry. I could not cry at home. The children needed me to be strong. Any sign of weakening on my part would have created incredible tension in their lives. They were young and needed to see their mother confident and cheerful. They had their own pressure and pain to bear. Growing up isn't easy either. So I couldn't cry at home or at the hospital. Merrill liked my courage. He respected the way I faced up to the most unpleasant tasks and did them without flinching. But all this stiff-upper-lipping was getting to me. I had bottled up my emotions and there was a torrent of tears trapped down inside me, waiting to be released. It happened one day when I least expected it.

Merrill's special nurse had been a great help to me. We had cleaned the burns together. We had learned to laugh and make it all a game—comparing the size and weight of the scabs we had pulled, joking about the ugliest of tasks. She was important to Merrill's healing and we needed her. One day the chief nurse's office announced that our special nurse was worn out and had requested a leave of absence. She was to be replaced by a senior student nurse.

I marched into the office and tried to explain why an inexperienced student nurse could not possibly be adequate for this crucial stage of Merrill's healing.

"I am sorry, Mrs. Womach, but the student we have assigned you is quite competent, and besides there is no other nurse available."

Suddenly I felt that long-stifled scream welling up inside me. I began shouting. "No experienced student is going to work on my husband," I yelled at her. "I don't want an amateur in the room. I want a trained professional."

I was throwing a tantrum. I ran into the hall and began to cry. Great uncontrolled sobs gasped up out of me. They were giving me a kid to work on my husband. It wasn't fair. The special nurse and I had been giving him strong doses of Demerol every day. We had to work like Trojans for hours to get the scabs pulled off. She would stand on one side, I on the other. My husband's new face was forming somewhere underneath those scabs. One bad treatment by an inexperienced nurse could mar the looks and slow the healing of the man I loved. So I wept angry tears.

I thought I was crying for him and for his face, but I was crying for me. I had been strong and silent long enough. It was time to cry, and I took advantage of it. Puddles of tears formed in the hall where I stood. The nurses walked by in embarrassed silence. Nothing would comfort me. I had bottled up all those feelings of anger and self-pity long enough. They needed to be released, and it felt good to cry them away. I had to let the cork out of the bottle and let my emotions go, or I could have had a nervous breakdown. After my cry I felt embarrassed and ashamed, until Dr. Hamacher and I had a long cup of coffee in the cafeteria.

"I'm sorry I cried, Dr. Hamacher," I blurted out, but he interrupted with a laugh.

"Virginia, it was the best thing in the world for you to cry that way," he said. "You needed it and you deserved it."

"But I yelled at the head nurse. I made a fool of myself."

"Nonsense," Hamacher said, "she understood perfectly well. She has watched you working with Merrill day after day. Both of us were worried about how you could hold up under all the new tasks and tensions with all your feelings bottled up. We were both relieved when you cried. It was just what you needed."

I had never thought of tears as a necessary part of the healing process. I had never seen anger as remedial. But without that wild, wonderful cry in the hall I am afraid those bottled tensions might have been terribly destructive in the long run.

The funny thing is that the student nurse was a wonderful person. She learned quickly and helped speed up, not slow down, my husband's healing. She turned out to be a precious young woman and friend. I learned to love and appreciate her very much. And through all of this I was becoming more and more aware of the incredible way God works to help us through our suffering and to bear all the pressures that come our way.

7

The Rebuilding Would Begin

FIFTY-ONE DAYS AFTER the flaming crash, Dr. Hamacher began the first of a series of skin graft operations that went on for eleven years. Plastic surgery is often misunderstood. Virginia told me before the surgery that my son, Dan, had been worried for days about the operations. Although the children were not allowed to visit me for weeks, Virginia kept them informed about my progress.

"What's the matter, son?" she asked him. "Plastic surgery will help Dad get well and bring him home again."

There was a long pause.

"I know, Mom," Dan said, "but he can never play baseball with me again."

"Why?" she questioned. "Of course he can."

"But he'll be plastic. He could break."

Apparently Dan was thinking of plastic picnic plates that bend and break easily. He didn't know how I would manage with such fragile, breakable skin. He didn't realize that my new skin was just old skin from another part of me grafted onto a burned area to replace skin destroyed in the fire.

The day before that first major surgery, Dr. Hamacher visited me to explain the process. It was necessary to lay down base skin across the entire surface of my face and the back sides of both hands. That skin would be removed from my chest with a Padgett Dermatome. He sat in a chair near my bed and unwrapped a small green package.

"The dermatome is wrapped this way, Merrill, to keep it sterile and after I show you how it works it will have to be sterilized again. We go to a lot of work to keep you from getting an infection."

The little machine looked like an old semicircular, rolling ink blotter with a knife attached.

"We cover the round surface with glue," he explained. "Your skin adheres to the glue and as we roll the surface upward the knife travels down along the surface, cutting free a split thickness of skin twelve- to fifteen-thousandths of an inch thick. The sheet of skin retrieved can be as small as three by eight inches or as large as four by sixteen inches. The skin is then carefully attached to the damaged area with sutures or threads."

Virginia and the nurses had spent weeks preparing the burn areas to receive the new skin. This was an exciting moment for me, like being born again piece by piece. I had no face. Everything was burned away. Soon I would have my face again. Soon I could leave the hospital and get back to my family and my business.

The doctor interrupted my dream.

"Merrill, these are difficult operations. I am not a magician. I cannot take you in like a burned pumpkin and send you out days later looking like you looked before. We have limited skin to work with. Your forehead is one kind of skin. The eyebrows are another kind with hair. Your nose is skin with sebaceous material in it. Your chin is not. Now all those delicately balanced, very different skin types will be replaced with a sheet of skin from your chest. Later we will try to find appropriate skin to graft into special areas. We will try to rebuild your eyelids with hair-bearing skin and your nose without it, but we are human and we are limited. You must not dream too great a dream or you will end up disappointed."

I interrupted him.

"Why are you telling me all these things?"

"Yesterday," he answered, "I performed a serious operation on a three-year-old child with a large blood-vessel tumor. His mother called me to ask if she could carry the child down into surgery. I asked her, 'Why do you want to steal from your son?' I tried to explain to her that even little children need to learn how to handle stress. 'If you carry your son into surgery, if you handle his stress for him, when will he learn to face suffering on his own?'

"She stared at me for the longest time. Her eyes filled with tears. Then she nodded, slowly, silently and walked away. The next morning I watched her kiss her little child in his room, and when she turned to leave he screamed and hollered for her. She froze in place for a moment, weighing her response, then turned slowly and said, 'Son, climb up on the carriage. The doctor will help you. I'll be waiting right here for you.' Then she turned and left the room.

"For a moment he hollered again, reaching out to his departing mother. Then he stopped, looked up at us, and climbed up on that carriage as brave as you please. On the way to surgery he looked up and down the hall, asked questions in the elevator and smiled at the anesthesiologist. His mother didn't steal that proud, brave moment from her child by clinging to him. She let him face suffering and he faced it well.

"Merrill," Dr. Hamacher continued, "I have decided that my patients should have a chance to know and understand what is going on, so they can face it. Taking the mystery out of medicine often takes the fear out as well. Knowing means the patient can prepare for whatever lies ahead, instead of being surprised by it. It is a risk to bring you into the process, but I believe it is a greater risk to leave you out."

After Dr. Hamacher left the room I had a strange sense of well-being. My dreams for a handsome new face (or even my moderately handsome old one) had been corrected from the beginning. My mind whirled with new information: *dermatomes, split-thickness grafts,* and *nonabsorbing sutures.* But I felt glad that he had told me and better prepared for whatever would happen that next day in surgery.

Hamacher was a master of timing. After many long weeks without a visit from my children, he had arranged it for today. I missed them so. We had spoken on the telephone, but my voice was strange and distorted. They had spoken to me from behind the closed door. They were polite, but found it difficult to believe that the person they never saw was really their dad. They could not enter the hospital room because, in my unstable, open-wound condition, any little infection they might carry could be fatal to me.

The doctor had suggested that the children stand across the street from the hospital five floors down and wave at me through the window, and regularly Virginia would bundle them up and stand on the corner waiting for nurses to wheel me to the window for a brief time of waving and blowing kisses. Needless to say, this did not substitute for holding them in my arms. They looked up and saw a strange and distant figure. The day came when I would see them at last! My head was like raw meat. My beard grew through the open burns. I was still swollen and entirely unrecognizable.

*   *   *   *   *

I SPENT MANY DAYS preparing our children for this first visit to Merrill's hospital room. They had waited a long time to see their father and were beginning to wonder if someone else was playing Merrill at that window. They were beginning to fear that their father had died in the plane crash and that we were just pretending he was still alive. I still vividly remembered that first time I saw him in the hospital in Klamath Falls and the shock and nausea that I felt. So I tried to get them ready. In fact, I'm afraid I overprepared them.

One of Merrill's friends had visited him recently—with disastrous results. She entered the room, took one look at him, turned white, and almost fainted. Merrill was concerned for her and asked, "Kathy, are you all right?" Her voice pitched up two or three octaves and squeaked, "Of course I'm all right. Why wouldn't I be all right?"

Then she started talking ninety miles an hour. "I'm fine," she insisted. "What makes you think I'm not all right?" With that, she walked out into the corridor and began to cry. She couldn't sleep for days after seeing him. I didn't want the children to suffer the same kind of shock and embarrassment, so I bought a roast and unwrapped it in the kitchen. The raw meat was oozing blood.

"That is the way Daddy's face looks," I said, "and his hands look the same." I squeezed the roast to make the blood drip as Merrill's blood dripped onto the pillow and bed sheets. By the time I was through with my little Alfred Hitchcock special, they looked back and forth in wide-eyed wonder.

I didn't want their reactions to hurt or embarrass Merrill, either, but the oversized surgical smocks, caps, and masks they had to wear would hide their reactions from him. Only their eyes showed between the caps and the masks as we entered the room that day.

I told them just before entering that if they felt faint or wanted to leave to stand by me and squeeze my hand. I would then take them from the room as if nothing was the matter. Our plan was ready. The preparations had been made, but when we entered the room and they knew at last that their daddy really was alive, all the ugly burns in the world couldn't keep them from him.

They clustered around his bed, giggling and telling crazy jokes, catching him up on the neighborhood gossip, and asking him about the accident and the surgery that lay ahead. Nobody squeezed my hand that day. They were incredibly brave and enthusiastic and unshockable. Dan walked right over to the bed.

He was barely tall enough to look above the rail. His wide eyes were the only part of him that Merrill could see. But his eyes flashed love and joy, and Merrill got the message all three of the children were sending him: "We love you, Daddy. It doesn't matter how you look. We're glad you are alive." No medicine could have done for Merrill what those three troopers did in that first brief visit.

*   *   *   *   *

THE NEXT MORNING as the nurses prepared me for surgery, I could still see Judie, Marlene, and Danny peering happily at me from behind those surgical masks. I felt happy as the orderly wheeled me down the hospital hall and onto the elevator. A nurse took over as the operating-room doors slid open to receive me. I was transferred to the operating table and lay there looking up into a panel of soft white light. Now the rebuilding would begin. Now my life was in the hands of Dr. Hamacher and his dermatome machine, his split-thickness grafts, and his sutures.

He came humming into the operating room. His voice boomed out, "Hi, sport, how are you today?" A string of jokes followed his greeting until the operation theater rang with laughter. In the many surgeries that followed during the next twelve years, I cannot remember the time he didn't come whistling or singing up the hall, his cigar smoldering, his heavy heels thumping down the hallway. And always he had new jokes. Right in the middle of taking stitches out of my face, he would tell a joke. I would strain not to laugh, not to move while he was pulling out the stitches. But invariably his good humor would win out and the work had to stop while the laughter rang. The last thing I remembered before surgery was his laughter. Perhaps some complained, but I felt healing in that laugh.

When I awakened after surgery, I was in my room again, and

only Virginia's firm hand kept me from crawling to that mirror
to see Dr. Hamacher's handiwork.

"How do I look, Virginia?" I asked.

"You look like a pile of wet gauze," she answered.

"I was hoping I had my face back."

"You do," boomed Hamacher, just entering the room, "or a
second chest with ears," he laughed. He had removed a large
piece of skin from my chest and fastened it across my face.

For two weeks I lay wrapped like a mummy, my face covered
with tight, Ace bandages. Two tubes stuck through the elastic
casing into my nose. Virginia used a giant syringe to suck up
liquid-protein dinners and squeeze this milk-shake type sub-
stance down through the tubes into my stomach.

The sheet of newly grafted skin had been sutured to the
fleshy granules below—by over five hundred little stitches. As
we waited for the donor area to heal and grow, I felt more
and more trapped inside those bandages. I couldn't see. It
was difficult to hear. The tubes irritated and clogged my
breathing. I was getting a severe case of claustrophobia. Finally, after fourteen days Dr. Hamacher carefully peeled away
the bandages and premiered my new face to Virginia and the
nurses. The transplant had not taken hold yet and in less than
sixty seconds the bandages were in place again. But in that
minute Virginia had a terrible shock.

Later I learned from one of the nurses that the sheet of transplanted skin was white and ghostly. My new face looked dead and
shapeless. There was only one slit for the right eye to peer
through, and no natural features. Virginia later confessed that
the first look left her weak with horror. Ten days later Dr. Hamacher took off the bandages again.

"Beautiful," he whispered to himself, "just beautiful."

My left eye was closed over by the grafted skin. There was a
little slit for my right eye to peer through. I blinked nervously,
trying to open it wider.

"That is all you will see for a while, Merrill," Dr. Hamacher explained. "I just wanted you to be able to see enough to get around your home."

"I'm going home?"

"That's right," he answered. "Just as soon as this new graft looks like it will hold. This isn't the end, Merrill," he warned. "We've just begun, but you need a rest, and some time with your family in your own home will do you good."

That new graft was beginning to cause me a great deal of discomfort as the anesthetic wore off and I could feel the blood pumping in my face and hands. I felt bad but I looked even worse. The grafted skin went straight across my face from cheek to cheek. There was no bridge for a nose, just two slits for nostrils. My lips were pulled completely open, exposing my gums and teeth. There was no adequate way to close my mouth and I could hardly see through the little peephole in the new mask of skin I wore.

My hands were in no better condition. They were blood-red and throbbing. They were still stiff and clawlike. My fingers were stuck together by the oozings. I lay back in disappointment and remembered Hamacher's words. I had been warned. It would not happen overnight. A piece of skin, four-by-eight inches, fifteen-thousandths of an inch thick, had been removed by a dermatome from my anterior chest wall and attached to the damaged area with nonabsorbable sutures. It was only a foundation, but I was going home. At least for a few weeks I would sleep in my own bed again.

It was an exciting thought, yet that hospital room had become a very secure world for me. I was glad to leave it and yet I was a bit nervous at the prospect of being away from all the equipment and personnel available in that place. I had spent many hours there, with my brothers and sisters, our larger family, and my friends gathered around the bed. Dwayne and Wayne, my friends and fellow workers in National Music Service, had done

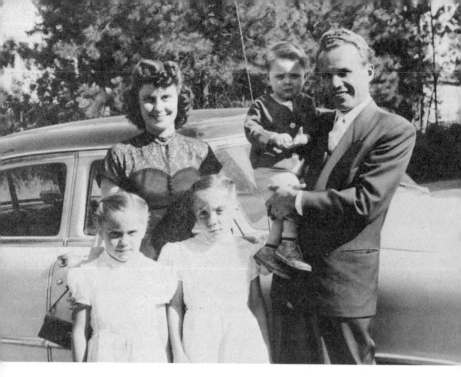

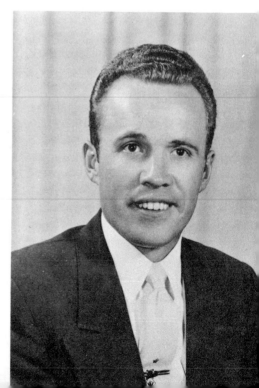

The Womachs on the way to church in 1955. *Left to right:* Marlene, Virginia, Judie, Dan, Merrill. *Right:* Merrill, a year before the 1961 crash.

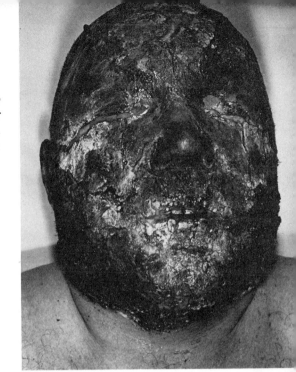

Merrill after the crash. Photo by Dr. Hamacher. *Below: Crash site thirteen years later. Photo by Mel White Productions.*

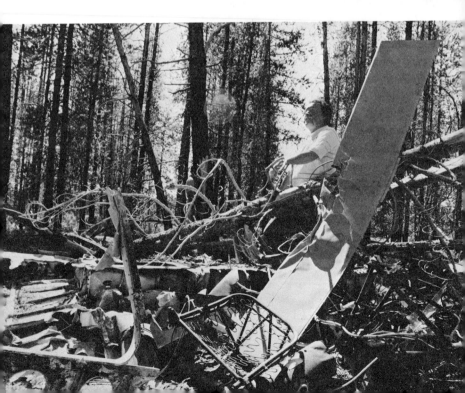

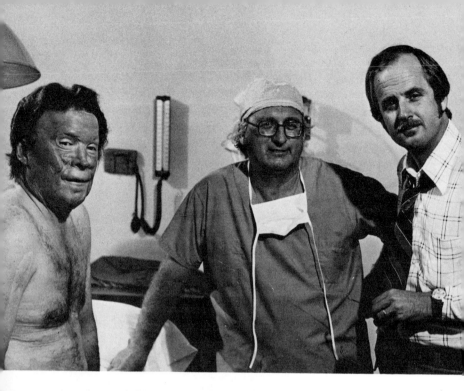

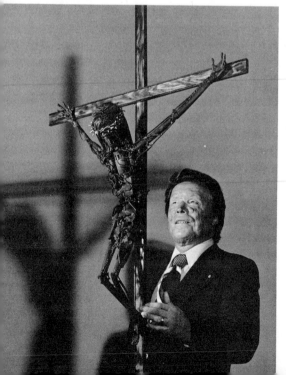

Hospital revisited. *Left to right:* Merrill, Dr. Hamacher, Mel White. *Photo by Mel White Productions.* *Left:* Merrill with sculpture made from wreckage. *Photo by Mel White Productions.*

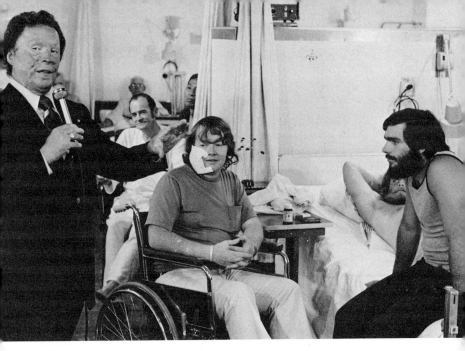

Entertaining at Veterans Hospital, Spokane. *Photo by Mel White Productions. Below:* The Womachs at home. *Photo by Mel White Productions.*

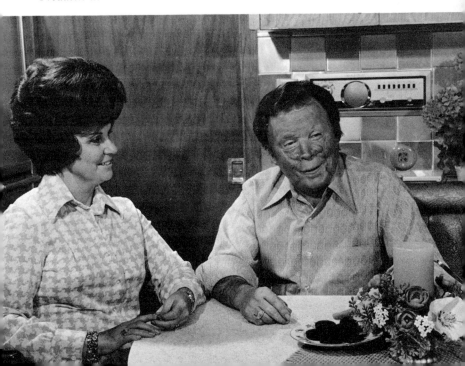

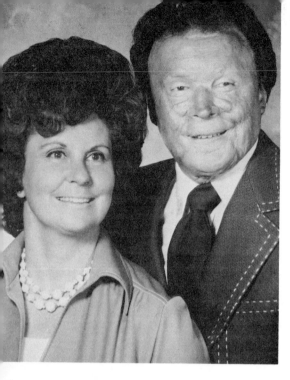

Strength in the sharing: Virginia and Merrill. *Below:* Family group. *Seated (left to right):* Merrill, Benny Cook, Shanna Sowards, Virginia. *Standing (left to right):* Ben and Marlene Cook, Dan and Cathryn Womach, Judie (holding Ryan) and Phil Sowards.

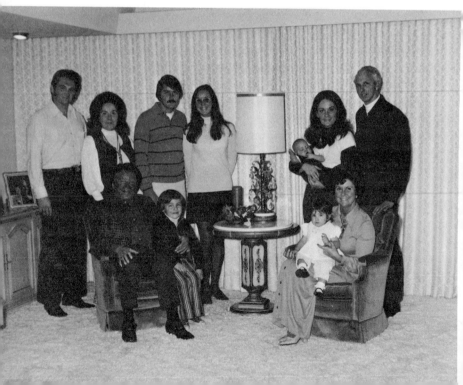

8

God's Plan Is Best

FOR SEVENTY DAYS and nights Merrill had lain in hospital beds, suffering excruciating pain from the burns on his face and hands before plastic surgery could begin. I watched the nurses on their nighttime rounds giving him large doses of painkiller to help him sleep. In the daytime, before each scab-pulling treatment, nurses gave him more shots to ease the pain. Soon Merrill was going home. For months ahead the sheets would still run with blood. Scabs would have to be painfully pulled and the new grafted and donor areas would throb day and night without letup. He felt he needed those painkillers, and yet Dr. Hamacher was determined to prevent another case of hospital drug addiction.

One morning he and Merrill were discussing the transition from hospital to home care. "There is a trained nurse living just across the street from us," Merrill told the doctor. "She can give me shots when I need them."

Hamacher sat down near Merrill's bed. "Merrill, I want you to do one thing," he said. "Get a contractor to build a room in the middle of your house. Put the phone in there and a toilet and one small window that will allow Virginia to pass food and messages to you. Then we will call the nurse from across the street, and she can come and give you shots whenever you need them."

Abruptly he stood and left the room. Both of us were silent. Dr. Hamacher had seen too many good people become drug addicts during long hospital stays. He had watched too many families destroyed, lives ruined, and homes broken because the painkilling habit was not caught in time. He was determined that it not happen to Merrill.

Merrill was not addicted, yet he really needed those shots before each painful treatment. Merrill used to sit by the window and wait for Hamacher's car to appear in the lot below. When Hamacher arrived to make his rounds, to remove the sutures, or to pick and to probe, Merrill would quickly call a nurse and get his shot before Hamacher walked through the door. One morning Merrill sat watching the parking lot when Hamacher surprised him and walked in the door.

"Hey, what are you doing here?" he asked. "Your car isn't down there, is it?"

Hamacher mischievously played innocent. "I got a new car, Merrill. Why do you ask?"

"Oh, it isn't important," he said. "I just kind of hoped to have a warning before you began to torture me so that. . . ." His voice trailed off.

"So that you could get your shot?" Hamacher cut in.

Merrill nodded like a schoolboy caught in the middle of a childish prank. Hamacher called in the nurse and walked over to Merrill holding her injection needle.

"I told you, Merrill, that as long as you needed these shots you would get them. But I also said that the day would come when you wouldn't need them anymore, and I promised on that day I would not let you have them anymore. That day came fourteen days ago."

Hamacher squeezed the contents of the needle onto the floor. "You've been getting sterile-water shots for about two weeks," he said, "and you didn't have any idea. Right?"

Both of the men stood there smiling at each other. Hamacher continued, "Painkillers are for psychological help as well as for physical pain. If we give you a shot and promise you another one in four hours, by the fourth hour you will be screaming for that shot whether you need it for pain, or think you need it. We can make hospital addicts through this process. God gave us drugs to alleviate pain, and we make addicts."

*   *   *   *   *

THE DAY I MET DR. HAMACHER he asked me if I took sleeping pills or pain pills or even aspirin regularly. I thought it a strange question then. The day I left the hospital he reminded me that I had answered *no* to all counts. In a parting shot he said, "Womach, if you take even one aspirin in the next five weeks you can get yourself another doctor." Then he walked out into the hallway and said something to Virginia before he disappeared on his hospital rounds.

"What did Dr. Hamacher say, Virginia?" I asked as she came in the door.

She looked stunned and surprised by his words. She quoted them back to me. "Virginia," he had said, "years from now when I meet Merrill on the street I want to shake his hand and know that he's not an addict because I allowed him to be."

*   *   *   *   *

THAT DAY WAS MERRILL'S birthday—February 7. Exactly seventy-six days after he had crashed he was coming home at last. Merrill had already pulled on his trousers, but the nurse had been instructed to give him one last shot to help him survive the painful trip to our home in North Spokane. They had placed silk dressings over his donor areas and had his pajamas over the silks so they would not stick to his trousers. The donor area was still oozing. He put his pants on over the pajamas.

By the time Merrill had been through this long process of getting dressed, he was dripping wet with sweat. He had not moved for many weeks. He was weak because he hadn't been exercising and was glad to sink into the wheelchair and be wheeled through the hospital towards our station wagon parked below. Nurses, doctors, orderlies, and staff greeted us along the way. They knew he would be back again and again. They knew the surgeries had just begun, but we were going home and they all wished us well.

Merrill climbed into the car and lay exhausted on the seat. "Honey," his voice was barely audible, "could you stop by the office on our way home, please?"

He was quite a sight—staggering slowly into that office, greeting our little staff, and sitting down at his desk after too long an absence, but it was easily apparent that he should be home in bed. Dwayne helped me get Merrill back into the car and we drove the last few miles to our home. It was strange how people would pull up alongside our car, take a glance at Merrill, then look back again the second time to see what kind of monster was sitting there.

He had bandages all around his face. Try to bandage a round head and have the mouth and eyes and nostrils still free. It is quite a challenge and leaves the person beneath the gauze looking rather abnormal. By now the gauze wrappings on his face and hands were dripping with blood, slime, and sweat. The donor area, too, was sticky because the scab had gotten wet from Merrill's perspiration. When he tried to get into bed, his trousers would not come off. They stuck to him. We had to soak his pajamas off in the bathtub before we could change them and get him into bed. After that episode it was a long time before Merrill tried to do so much in one quick trip again.

Those first days at home were really awful for the whole family. Merrill had just come off the drugs and his pain was severe. He was nervous and high-strung. It was hard for him to cope with the pain at first because he was used to getting help when he needed it at the hospital. When we got home, all medicine was stopped, so it was hard for him to be able to do things to keep his mind occupied. Many times the whole family had to walk very gingerly. He got upset at the smallest noise. If the children were fighting, he could hardly stand it. At first he was very agitated, and we just tried to keep out of his way.

* * * * *

IT WAS VERY DIFFICULT for me to get used to being home again. There is security in the hospital. You are in one room and there are professionals there day and night watching out for your needs, guaranteeing your health and safety. But when I arrived home, I felt helpless. Every time the gas heater came on, I saw myself in the flames in my exploding airplane. I could see them and feel them burning away my face. In the middle of the night I would wake up suddenly when the heater came on, terrified that the house was on fire. I was worried about Virginia and the children and their safety. I was the man of the house and if there were any kind of crisis, I would be helpless to save them. I couldn't do anything. I couldn't see. I had no strength or energy. I am a proud and independent man, and that feeling of helplessness made me angry and difficult to live with, I am sure.

Also, I had nightmares every night. Not having any kind of painkiller made sleeping very difficult. So I tossed and turned through the long night hours in that restless half-sleep. My mind dreamed wildly. The dreams were strange, even funny in their symbolism. Two I remember occurred often.

I dreamed I was going along an old, rocky, bumpy road in the back of a cart being drawn by a horse. The cart was filled with people. I was lying down and there was a little dark-haired boy, ten or twelve years old, picking the scabs off my face with a big machete. Every time the cart hit a bump the machete would cut deep and painfully into my face. He cut and jabbed me the entire journey.

Another nightmare is difficult for me to recall today without feeling sick to my stomach. I was out on a long, green football field, kicking a football around with my family and several dear friends. Suddenly we were surrounded by people trying to catch

us and tie our hands behind our backs. There was a huge oven
at the end of the field. We waited in a line that moved slowly
toward the flaming oven. As we got closer I could see that the
enemy was throwing each of my friends and family into that oven
one by one and baking them until they were burned and bloody.
As the people were pulled back out of the oven they were screaming in pain and horror. As they were carried past, I could see that
their faces were burned away. Their hands were bloody claws.
Each of the people looked like me.

I went home in February, and at that time Indian astrologers
were predicting that a planet would hit the earth. I didn't believe
it, but I began to worry. The cold war with Russia was escalating,
and that also caused me to worry. As I withdrew from painkilling
drugs, my mind whirled. I still had great pain and couldn't sleep
or dozed restlessly. Pictures of bombings, invasions, fiery planets
striking the earth, and even fantasies about our furnace blowing
up and our house burning down plagued me in those long, restless nights. If some catastrophe would strike us, I would be helpless. What if my family needed me? I could not see. I could hardly
walk. I had no strength. My body was a mass of painful, healing
wounds. I was not worried for myself, but for them I was husband
and father and I was useless.

*   *   *   *   *

MERRILL WOULD AWAKEN ME in the middle of the night, afraid
that the house was on fire. I would help him out of bed and we
would make a slow, painful tour through our home, checking
on the children, checking the furnace and the gas heaters and
major appliances. He had to be sure everything was all right
before he could go back to bed again. It was pitiful to watch
him groping through the darkness, peering through the one
small slit in his grafted face. He had no nose and no eyebrows.
The skin gaped open at his mouth, and teeth and gums pro-
truded. His bedclothes often ran with blood and slime so badly

that we would change the sheets several times in the night. He was in such pain, but still I had to continue tearing away those scabs with forceps, keeping the damaged areas from growing over, preparing them to receive new skin grafts in the operations that lay ahead.

The donor areas where large sheets of skin had been removed from his buttocks were especially painful. We had to buy boxer shorts and cut out large circles to permit the air to circulate and keep cloth out of the healing wounds. The new scabs were more than an inch thick. When Merrill moved, often eight or ten inches of scab would tear open and bleed again. He deeply suffered from the pain and inconvenience of these running, bleeding sores.

We had a hospital bed in the house and I was an old pro at changing it by this time. I had often changed his bedclothes in the hospital. Nurses were often too busy and I had learned the ropes. I had the house ready to serve as Merrill's hospital. We had stacks of sheets and pillowcases and bed dividers. At one time after the accident Merrill dropped in weight to ninety-seven pounds. He was simply bleeding to death. They were giving him drugs to thin his blood, and so the open burns just constantly oozed saline from his body. When I married him he had a beautiful body, a strong physique. His chest and upper arms were large and muscular. He had a good torso. But after the accident and the constant bleeding he was nothing but skin and bones.

Merrill's brother John brought him an exercycle which his family had used when his daughter contracted polio. Merrill would struggle gamely to mount and ride that bike. At first he could only go a couple of rounds. Then he stretched it to the equivalent of a quarter of a mile. Little by little his strength increased: half a mile, a mile, ten miles, twenty miles. The pain of riding that exercycle was intense as his burn areas, tight and inflexible, were forced up and down. The donor areas, with their thin layer of skin removed for transplant, were open sores, sometimes ten inches long by six inches wide. His whole body was covered by tight scars or running wounds, yet he kept on riding that cycle, trying to rebuild his strength.

It wasn't an easy time for any of us. I was trying to keep the children happy and out of Merrill's way. If I sensed that an argument between the children was coming, I would lay down whatever I was doing, hurry them outside, and try to settle it peacefully. I was nurse and cook and housekeeper and orderly and custodian and night watchman and mother and wife. Merrill had his own painful struggles. He cared about me and my problems, but he had hardly enough strength to rebuild his own body and business. The children cared about their mother, too, but they were young and adolescent and their lives and problems were all they had strength to bear. It was a very lonely time.

I lay in bed at night peering over the bed divider at a man I could not recognize. I wanted him to love me, to kiss me, to hold me in his arms. And there he lay oozing and suffering great pain. I prayed for strength and tried to sleep. It was a hard time for both of us.

But even then we could see how God had helped prepare us for this moment. When our son, Danny, was a baby he contracted a bad case of pneumonia. He became more and more congested until he could hardly breathe. We rushed him to the hospital and sat watching him lying in that little oxygen tent struggling for life. At first I sat there in a daze. It was hard to believe that he was dying. Then I got angry. Danny was my last child. I could have no more. He was my only son and he was dying. Nurses rushed around Danny. I could see that he had turned purple. His breathing had stopped. I left the room as they worked to restore his breathing.

I began to pray desperate, angry prayers. "God, don't take my baby away from me." My fingers gripped Merrill's hand until my knuckles were white and achy. Danny got worse and my prayers got more desperate. "Don't do this to me," I prayed. The doctor removed mucus from Danny's mouth and nose. Little tubes I didn't understand gurgled in and out of my dying child. We walked the halls. Alone in the hospital women's room, I locked myself in a toilet stall and cried, "Don't let Danny die." I remember blowing my nose into the toilet paper and crying until my eyes were tired and swollen. "Please let my baby live!"

The hospital staff was doing all that could be done to save our son. There was nothing more we could do but wait. Merrill and I had a weekly radio broadcast "Songs in the Night" from a nearby church studio. Helpless to do more for Danny, we went quickly to the studio just in time to make our broadcast schedule. During the program Merrill shared our concern for little Danny and asked the listeners to join in prayer for our son. Then Merrill prayed a prayer I will never forget. He didn't beg God to heal Danny. He just said simply and quietly: "God, Danny is Your child, too. You gave him to us for these four months. We have been blessed by having him. We had great dreams for him, but if You want him back, Lord, he is Yours. Amen." Then Merrill put his arm around me. Tears streamed down his face as we returned to the hospital.

Everything was quiet as we walked back into Danny's hospital room. The baby's color had returned. His breathing was almost normal. The nurse smiled and patted me on the arm. Then she left us alone with our child. Danny was alive. One moment he was dying. The next he was well. We had surrendered him and our plans for him to God. Whatever happened now, we would be content. If we had entered that room and found our child dead, we would have been sad and angry and disappointed, but I believe that after those first waves of grief passed over we would have still felt as we feel today. God is alive and working in our lives. We told Him what we wanted. We shared with Him our dreams. Then we said, "God's plan is best."

Lying there beside my suffering husband, seeing him awakened by nightmares, turning and twisting in pain, it was hard to believe that "God's plan is best." But even then I knew it was true. God was still alive and He was still working in our lives. I had no idea where He was taking us. I had no sense of what lay ahead, but I could say and believe it as I rolled over and tried to sleep, "Lord, we want Your plan in our lives. Just give us the strength to make it through each new day until that day comes when we do understand."

9

Strength in the Sharing

EIGHT WEEKS AFTER a wide sheet of skin from my chest was grafted above my mouth from cheek to cheek, Dr. Hamacher made a grim discovery. The scar tissue below my mouth, covering the area of my chin and lower face, was very thick. My beard was still growing beneath this tight layer of scar tissue and the whiskers could not penetrate the hard burned flesh. I had ingrown hair all over my face, trapped under the sheets of scab. The trapped hair curled and grew hard like an S.O.S. pad. Now and then one sharp strand would penetrate the skin, leaving a bleeding boil. I could take tweezers and pull the long clumps of hair through the hole. My face was covered with these little sores through which strands of whiskers had grown. The pain and discomfort were mounting. Something had to be done.

I returned to the hospital and Dr. Hamacher peeled away the layers of scar tissue. He cut away the months of accumulated whiskers. Then each beard-growing follicle beneath the surface was removed. A graft of new skin had to be sliced from a donor area on my chest with the dermatome machine. Then the skin was sutured across my lower face. The ingrown-hair problem had been solved, but I would never shave again.

My new face felt hard and tight. Every time I moved, sharp pains made me aware of the inflexible mask of skin I wore. I never thought of skin before my accident. I was never aware of it. I could laugh and squint and yawn without discomfort. I could stand before large audiences and sing operatic arias or old gospel

83

songs and never feel any pain. I could back each dramatic passage with the appropriate facial expressions without an ounce of suffering. Never once before the accident do I remember feeling my face. Now I felt every facial move I made. Now I could not even close my eyes or speak or eat without feeling the painfully tight band of skin.

I began to wonder if I would ever sing freely again. God had spared my voice, but how could I ever step in front of an audience feeling bound up like a mummy! A singer communicates with his whole face, not just his voice. When people watched me sing before my accident, they felt the message of that song because my face and my voice were a team. Now half of the team was dead. I still sang. Often in the later surgeries under a local anesthetic I would sing from the operating table. I was not ungrateful. It was good to be alive. But I began to worry that even though my voice had not been damaged its container had been burned away.

Lying in that hospital bed, my mind never stopped. I worried and wondered and sometimes felt depressed. It happened especially after surgery during those half-awake-half-asleep recovery times when it was hard to resist depression. Would I ever sing before large audiences again? Would I ever feel the thrill of hearing a great orchestra playing an introduction to a song I soon would sing? Would I ever walk out from behind the curtains and move people with God's great gift of song? I sang in the hospital, but even as I sang I wondered if it would ever be the same again.

I also wondered about my family. Would I ever recover my strength fully? Would I ever be able to feel like a strong, able father or husband again? How would my family and my friends react to years of ugly scars and painful healing? During those endless hospital nights I wondered about everything from a Russian invasion to a planet striking the earth. And in the daylight hours the questions went on. What else could I do lying in the hospital room? There was only a narrow slit in the skin of my face through which my right eye peered. It was difficult or impossible to read. I could not watch television. I could make telephone calls but still felt cut off, isolated, and left behind. The hours seemed endless. I had been an active, aggressive man; now I felt like a vegetable growing in a hothouse.

While in college during the early years of my professional career, I sang in funeral services, along with many other public appearances. Sharing those hours of sadness with families of the deceased, I discovered how music could bring joy to a troubled spirit. I became aware of the valuable services which funeral homes perform for families in bereavement and I determined that I would develop a means to become part of a musical ministry to the bereaved.

In 1959 I began the National Music Service. I proposed to use my voice to minister to those in need by providing recorded music to funeral homes. My company would provide funeral homes with a full range of organ and vocal music on stereo cartridge tape. Musicians at funeral homes were not seen while they sang or played, so why not have the very best music on tape! Virginia and I set up a research and development program to design and build stereo cartridge player systems that would provide a live sound, free from any distortion and with perfect fidelity, along with worry-free service. I recorded songs for all kinds of funeral needs. Then I borrowed enough money to buy a little airplane and flew it up and down the West Coast, visiting funeral homes and talking to everyone who would listen.

During these early years I lived out of a suitcase. At first funeral directors found it difficult to believe that recorded music could minister to the bereaved. We risked everything to prove it. Since the musicians weren't seen anyway, why not tape? That way those songs could always have appropriate words easily understood and beautifully performed. So we engineered, manufactured, rehearsed, recorded, installed, and serviced our music system. There was little time to rest or relax. National Music Service was just getting off the ground when I crashed. For four years I had not stopped traveling up and down the land. Now suddenly I was flat on my back in a hospital bed. I could not work. I could not read. I could only lie and wait. I knew God was at work in my life, but what good could come from all these hours of lying flat on my back? What could God possibly bring out of all this needless suffering?

Little by little it dawned on me. In the quiet nighttime hours of the burn ward, my mind churned over the same questions time and time again. I was learning the hard way what it means to suffer. I was learning—the only real way one can—what people facing tragedy and pain must feel. I had comforted those who mourn. I had visited the sick or injured in many hospital rooms. I thought I understood their pain and loneliness. I had counseled or given words of encouragement, but not until I lay in the hospital myself did I know what it meant to toss and turn the night away. I discovered what it really felt like to lie awake and worry, to feel left out, passed by, and helpless. God was sensitizing me to suffering, as He could in no other way. Early in those long years of surgery I began to thank Him for this chance to experience this sad but necessary dimension to life. I would sing again, ugly scars or not, but my song would be different.

During those times others ministered to me. Virginia was an incredible source of strength. My family and friends were faithful. I can still see my children sneaking into my room, staring out from under those oversized surgical caps, carrying flowers picked from the garden and crazy cards they had designed. My mom and dad came often. My brothers and sisters sat in my room. My friends from our little company visited regularly. They all clustered around and tried to give me their best support.

Those visitors could not say much. They knew me. They knew what lying around was doing to me. They knew my pain and felt my worries, so they didn't speak. They just stood there and smiled or shared local gossip. So many people in the hospital are abandoned by family and friends who don't know what to do or say. Mine did just the opposite. They came and smiled and sat. I remember going to sleep under sedation, with Virginia and my brother John or Russell standing at my bedside. I would awaken a long time later and they would still be standing there. They were passing on their strength to me. They were praying, and their prayers were rebuilding my flagging spirit.

Other visitors were not so effective. I do not write these words easily or ungratefully. I write them because I think it is important to be honest. Many of my well-meaning Christian visitors caused more harm than good in their long visits to my bedside. Some of the very worst times I had in the hospital were during visits from concerned Christians who were trying to be helpful. Often their visits left me feeling miserable and depressed.

Visiting preachers were sometimes the most depressing. They would come into my room on the run. They would take one look at my face and go into shock. Their looks of grave concern left me feeling I should comfort them. Faking a smile, they would mumble, "God bless you, Merrill." I wanted to say something to give them hope, to cheer them up. They would chat for a moment. "We know how you feel, brother," they would mumble, and then ask to pray. I knew very well that they had no idea how I felt. But I could forgive them that because of all the hospital visits I had made, saying I understood, yet having no idea. It was the manner of their prayers which I found difficult to forgive. Many times those visiting clergymen would stand and pray for fifteen or twenty minutes. They would break down and sob. I thought they were feeling sorry for themselves. I felt they were crying about their own problems and using me as a kind of shock to get their tears rolling. I heard them asking God to heal me, but I could sense that they had little hope for that. I could hardly wait for their long mournful prayers to end. I felt like shouting at them, "Get it over with. Get out of here. Leave me alone. God knows what He is doing." But they meant well. So I said nothing.

Others would tell Virginia and me that we weren't praying right. "If you had more faith," they would scold us, "God would heal you. Pray in faith for God to heal you and He will make you just the way you were before." We had prayed. Thousands across the country had prayed. Letter-writing campaigns had been mounted to get those who knew me or who had heard me sing to pray for my healing and recovery. Dear friends were praying daily to that end. Virginia and I prayed, but once we had asked God—once we had made it plain—then we stopped struggling. We couldn't just keep yelling at God to make me well. We had to pray our way. One afternoon a friend came into the room and sat for a long time before he spoke.

"Merrill, we must not be praying right," he said, "or you would be healed. We must have more faith that God will make you well again."

Virginia said what we both believed. "We can't pray that way. God has put us through this for a purpose," she said. "He is doing this for a reason. We can't tell God what to do. We have to say, 'God, whatever You want to have happen to us, give us strength to be able to cope with it. Give us strength to take it in our stride. Whatever You have in store for us, we accept. Just help us bear it.' " Our friend didn't understand. Virginia's words did not break through to him. "We can't ask God to make Merrill just like he was before. God put us through this for a reason. We may not understand it yet, but we wouldn't miss His purpose for the world."

I really believe that, both then and now, Virginia and I are convinced that God could make my skin like a baby's again. He could give me back my original face and hands in an instant. But He has something else in mind. And even though we hate the pain and suffering and inconvenience and embarrassment, we want His will more than we want our own.

*   *   *   *   *

DURING MERRILL'S HOSPITALIZATION, we got some bizarre advice. People wrote letters that made me so upset I wouldn't even let Merrill see them after a while. Some would write us all kinds of thoughtless, crazy, inappropriate advice. They would claim that God had spoken to them about Merrill in a voice in the night. Or they would claim to have a prophecy about Merrill's healing. "All you have to do," one wrote, "is stand in the shower at midnight on Thursday next. Turn on the water. Put your face and hands into the water and God will wash all your scars away. He will make you completely new." They recommended other strange cures or foreign medicines or gifted healers. They all said that God had told them to tell us this or that nonsense. They all claimed to have special revelations for Merrill from God Himself, and they wrote and called and visited for years.

Merrill felt sorry for some of the insensitive clergymen who visited him. I have to confess that I sometimes felt let down by the church, too. Many people did not bring in food to help when I was running to the hospital and then back again. I made quick trips home to change clothes, to feed the kids, and to run them to school or their lessons. Then back to the hospital to be with Merrill. I cannot remember too many times in all those early months when Merrill was hospitalized that someone called or visited me or even offered to take the children to Sunday school. We talked to our pastor about it years later. He apologized and said what others have said and many probably felt. They thought everyone else was doing it, when few were doing anything at all. It seems that if you are really having problems and beg for help, church people come through, but until you beg they just don't get the message.

Still, the church *was* at work in our lives, since the church is people who love Christ and love their neighbor. One of the dearest friends I had through all those first overwhelming months lived right across the street from us. Pat Witham was the wife of an air-force noncommissioned career officer. She had three little children of her own, but when I was still in Klamath Falls with Merrill, I called her on the phone and explained my predicament. Judie and Marlene were with my mom and dad. My sister was keeping Danny. I thought I would be gone just a few days. I thought Merrill would be home in a week. But when I called Pat, she knew immediately what to do. She moved her three children over to our house, picked up my children, and cared for them all. She didn't want them to miss any school, so she didn't hesitate. She didn't call back and ask if she could help. She just moved in and set to work. She cooked and washed and cleaned. She took over the chores, and when I returned to Spokane she continued doing most of the housework, the cooking, and even chauffeuring the children so that I could spend my entire time with Merrill at the hospital.

Bill and Ruth Sperling were two other people who ministered in our lives during those awful first years. Merrill was sometimes depressed. He worried from time to time. He got angry and anxious periodically. His nerves flared up and he lost his temper now and then, but all through those bad times there was more singing than there was crying. But there was one time when Dr. Hamacher worked on the nerves in Merrill's hands. The nerve endings were exposed and every little contact made pain run up his arms like high-voltage electric shock. He couldn't touch the bed covers or lift a paper without feeling those exposed nerve endings. The skin was raw and still bloody. The grafts were tight and painful, and those raw nerve endings seemed to dangle, so that the slightest contact made him cry out in pain.

This gradually got Merrill into the most depressed state I had seen him. He spent two horrible, lonesome weeks after that operation. He could not get above it. Even music didn't make the difference. His depression grew daily. We had Christian friends drop by to visit. They would say, "Trust God and everything will be okay," and all their well-meaning advice just made him feel more and more angry and depressed. One of the strangest things about this particular down time was the way even Merrill's favorite Scripture verses, that had buoyed our spirit and made us feel better in the past, made him feel worse.

At first I tried to kid him out of it. I prepared food that he liked. I bought new records that would cheer him. Nothing worked. Then I began to feel depressed, too. I went down with him and felt what he was going through. The more we tried to read the Bible and pray and talk to others, the more depressed we got. It seemed that nothing could stop the slide deeper into depression.

Then a wonderful thing happened. One night Bill and Ruth Sperling dropped by for a late and unexpected visit. Merrill had played baseball with Bill and they had sung together in a barbershop quartet. Ruth and I had been together as coffee-drinking friends for many years. The Sperlings had gone to bed early that night because Bill had to leave on a trip the next morning at five o'clock. As they were lying in bed about to go to sleep, Bill suddenly sat up on the edge of the bed. "Let's go visit Merrill and Virginia," he said, and Ruth responded without hesitation, "Let's do that."

They dressed, got in the car, and drove across town to our house. When they rang our doorbell, Merrill was pacing around a metal kitchen chair he had placed on the living room carpet. He had not slept well for weeks. His entire body throbbed with pain from his burns and the open donor areas. The nerves in his hands sent sharp excruciating pains throughout his body upon the slightest contact. He paced the floor, unable to sit or stand. He was totally depressed. Several times he had wondered aloud if he shouldn't just get into the car and drive it over the Monroe Street Bridge. To plunge into the water, hundreds of feet below, and die would bring an end to the pain and suffering. I was helpless —so I paced with him in silence.

Opening the door, I couldn't have been more surprised to see Bill and Ruth standing there in the middle of the night smiling sheepishly. Bill said, "Virginia, I know this is crazy. Forgive us for getting you up but we just got an urge to visit you." Ruth confessed that they had driven past the house several times, feeling absolutely insane about waking us up, but they acted on their urge—and what a difference their visit made.

They didn't say, "How are you feeling?" They didn't mumble a few religious phrases and ask to pray. They came in giggling and feeling silly for awakening us. They put on the coffeepot and broke open a bag of old cookies they bought at an all-night market on the way. They talked about the baseball team and all the games Merrill and Bill had won, and moaned over the games they had lost. They sang duets from the old quartets they had learned—without the other parts. The harmony was flat and dissonant, but in those few, short, friendly hours they brought us back up out of our desolation. Their spontaneous visit broke all the rules, but before they left that night, the depression was gone. We were alive again.

Bill told us later what he had told his wife that evening as he lay in bed wondering if they should go to all the trouble to make that late night visit. "Ruth," he said, "the Lord is telling me I have to go to Merrill and talk to him. I don't know why." We knew why. God was taking care of us through Bill and Ruth. God heard our prayer and sent us friends to break depression's hold on us. As we shared happy memories and sad, as we laughed and cried, God reached down and lifted us up again. In the sharing there was strength.

10

I Know He Holds My Hand

AT FIRST MY HANDS were fixed in place like claws. The flesh had been burned away. The nerves were painfully exposed. The pads of each finger were gone. Before the accident I used to spend hours playing the piano and singing. When I came home from surgery I was determined to play the piano again. I had been away from it for six months. So I went to our little spinet piano in the living room, put my fingers gingerly on the keys, and tried to strike a chord. Pain rushed through my fingers and from them throbbed into my whole body. I could not push my fingers against the keys hard enough to make a sound.

I sat staring at that piano for days. I would look at the keys, then at my hands again. They were useless. They moved but they had no strength. Every day Virginia would bathe each finger. Carefully she would wash away the oozings and pick off the hardening scabs. At first the fingers grew together. My hands were becoming webbed, and Virginia worked to keep the fingers separate and healing. I exercised my fingers one at a time. I pressed against the keys, but the pain made playing impossible. How would I ever play again? Then one day I remembered how. An organ took very little pressure to play. I rushed to the phone and called Fred Murphy, an organ dealer in Spokane, who knew of the accident. When I asked to rent an organ he refused. "No, Merrill, I can't rent you an organ, but I will lend you one without cost as long as you need it."

He knew that Virginia and I were struggling to keep our company going. The two men who worked with us were technical people and unfamiliar with sales work. I was phoning across the country from my hospital bed, explaining to mortuary directors what National Music Service could provide, and Chris and Wayne were making some sales calls, but those days were tight and Fred Murphy's offer seemed too good to be true.

The next day a delivery truck arrived. Fred set up the organ and explained to me the way to play it. Then he stood back and pointed at the keyboard. "Okay, Merrill, play!" I looked down at my claws. Neither one of us believed that I would ever play again, but I sat down at the organ and began to play simple chords. The music filled our living room. I had to sing.

> O Lord my God, when I in awesome wonder
> Consider all the worlds Thy hands have made,
> I see the stars, I hear the rolling thunder,
> Thy pow'r thru-out the universe displayed!
>
> Then sings my soul, my Savior God, to Thee;
> How great Thou art, how great Thou art. . . .

*   *   *   *   *

I WAS IN THE KITCHEN when Merrill began to play again. I rushed to the living room. Tears rolled down my cheeks as I watched my husband playing that first song on Fred Murphy's electronic organ. Merrill's face was still just a bumpy layer of skin. He could hardly see through the one eye slit in the surface. His nose had no bone for a bridge. His mouth was just an opening in the mask. His neck was tight and forced his face down into his chest. His hair was beginning to grow back through the scars. His hands were bent and tight. But he was playing again.

I called Dr. Hamacher and told him the good news. There was a long silence on his end of the line. Dr. Hamacher wanted so badly for Merrill to be able to sing publicly again. He had never seen facial burns more serious than Merrill's; yet he knew how important it was for Merrill to regain freedom of movement and expression in his face again. Merrill had to smile. He had so much to tell the world through song and Dr. Hamacher wanted desperately to rebuild Merrill's face to the point where he could use it to communicate again. In the background Hamacher could hear Merrill's music, "O Lord my God. . . . How great Thou art." It was another sign to both of us that Merrill would stand before audiences again one day and sing about the God he loved and wanted to serve in song. In Hamacher's office late that day, he reminded Merrill that one day he should go out and sing publicly again. Neither of us dreamed that Merrill would take his advice so quickly.

The fourth week out of the hospital Merrill accepted an offer from our church to do an evening concert for them. Dr. Hamacher and I both thought it was too early. People would be shocked and surprised that he would try to sing publicly in such condition, but we did not protest. We knew that some people would be horrified and even made ill by his presence. It is difficult to describe how he looked. Most of them had not seen him since the accident. I had visited the church to give them reports from time to time. They even fixed a telephone line from Merrill's hospital room to the church sanctuary so that the whole congregation could hear his voice again, but few knew how bad he looked. His face was gone, and in its place was sewn a sheet of grafted skin with appropriate gaps through which to breathe and speak. Now he proposed to stand before that congregation and sing.

Merrill's hands trembled slightly as we walked toward the church that fourth Sunday. He was so weak that it was difficult for

him to walk without wobbling. His hands were wrapped. His
donor areas were tight. He made strange, gasping sounds as he
breathed through the rough, open nostrils. His mouth was pulled
open and revealed his gums and teeth. He looked awful, but he
entered that church as though he had never been burned. People
saw Merrill coming and rushed to welcome him. They were
shocked and surprised, but most of them got through those first
awkward moments. One woman complained loudly, "A man in
his condition has no right to come to church and make us ill," but
most everyone else seemed truly glad to have him back again.

When Merrill stood to sing, a quiet gasp spread in unison
across the church. People were shocked and horrified, as we had
feared. Then Merrill began to sing those old familiar words:

I Know Who Holds Tomorrow*

I don't know about tomorrow, I just live from day to day.
I don't borrow from its sunshine, for its skies may turn to
  gray.
I don't worry o'er the future, for I know what Jesus said,
And today I'll walk beside Him, for He knows what lies
  ahead.

By the time he got to that first chorus, the mood had entirely
changed. People who sat in shock and horror at what they saw
before them felt embarrassed that they had so reacted to the
surface changes in Merrill's life. Tears of gratitude began to roll.
Merrill had not changed. He was still there behind those burns.

Many things about tomorrow I don't seem to understand,
But I know who holds tomorrow, and I know He holds my
  hand.

I looked at Merrill's hands and thought of all those treatments
necessary to keep his fingers from growing together. We could
never have done it without God's strength in us. Merrill began

to sing the second verse. He had not rehearsed the words, so both of us were caught off guard as they came singing out of him:

I don't know about tomorrow, it may bring me poverty,
But the One who feeds the sparrow is the One who stands
by me.
And the path that be my portion may be through the
flame or flood. . . .

He couldn't finish the last line: "But His presence goes before me and I'm covered with His blood."*

*I KNOW WHO HOLDS TOMORROW Copyright 1950 by Singspiration, Inc. All rights reserved. Used by permission.

He just stood there, his face tucked down into his chest, his mouth held open in that kind of forced, sad smile. He was thinking of those flames eating away his face and hands. He was reliving that moment the seat belt would not open. He recalled the surge of Someone's power which tore it off and got him from the flaming wreckage. God had been with him through the flames. Merrill's tears that night were not tears of sadness or disappointment, but tears of gratitude and praise. No one spoke. No one moved. Merrill paused and then began to sing again:

Many things about tomorrow I don't seem to understand,
But I know who holds tomorrow, and I know He holds my
hand.

Merrill sang for more than an hour after that. When he finished, the entire congregation stood to their feet applauding. They were moved by Merrill's courage and were applauding him that night, but they were also saying thanks to God for bringing him back and for giving him a song again.

*   *   *   *   *

I STOOD BEFORE THAT congregation and knew that the song God had given me after the accident was different from the song before. I had sung about passing "through flame and flood" hundreds of times and in as many places, but never had that song meant so much to me. Great Christian hymns came to life, now that I was really dependent on God. I had never *really* suffered before, so I didn't understand. I sang about man's need for God's mercy and I had everything. Now I knew how it felt to have nothing—to be scared and lonely and in pain. Now I knew how waves of depression can knock you down again and again until you quit wanting to struggle against them. Now I knew how it felt to be ugly and to have people stare at me in horror. Now I knew how it felt to be helpless and how God was working to get me through. Now I understood—and those who listened could feel the difference.

Those old hymns and gospel songs meant much more to me during the long years of surgery because I could relate to them in an entirely different way. Many of them were songs of praise written in the midst of suffering. Now I understood how it feels to wonder and worry and even doubt, while at the same time feeling confident and grateful. Many times in those early years of surgery I would sit down to practice a song thanking God for His blessings, while my hands cried out in pain and my face bled and cracked as I sang. Still I could sing, "O Lord my God. . . . How great Thou art," and mean it.

After that first concert, Dr. Hamacher began a surgical program to free my hands and face to function as they had before the accident. It would be long and painful and difficult. Heavy scars had formed and needed to be removed. Granules of new flesh were growing in the burn areas, yet sheets of skin had to be cut off my chest and back and grafted on the areas not able to heal themselves. Thousands of hours of therapy were prescribed to get my muscles stretched and my nerves normal again. There were many problems. Some of them may seem small and insignificant on the surface. For example, my eyelids and eyelashes had been burned away. The day or two after I got out of the hospital it rained hard in Spokane. When I got out in that rain for the first time, it felt like someone were sticking pins in my eyeballs. The little drops of rain, which the eyelashes normally catch and the eyelids normally blink away, were hitting right on the surface of the eye. Dust created the same kind of problem when it wasn't raining. Any dirt or pollen in the air would sail right past the missing lids and lashes and land on the surface of the eye. Then, without the lids to wash the eyes clean, I had to wipe away the intruders with a handkerchief. My eyes still run, day and night, and the debris collecting in them must be wiped away.

Some of the problems created humorous though pathetic incidents. Dr. Hamacher wanted to rebuild my eyebrows. So he took hair-bearing skin and transplanted little gardens of hair above each eye. The object was to create eyebrows that would at least trap some of the rain and foreign particles that would otherwise fall directly on my eye. After a few weeks the new eyebrows would begin to pull free from where they were grafted. I could feel them breaking loose. They hung there half-attached, flopping around as I walked or turned my head. These hair-bearing skin patches needed cleaning two times a day. I knew I could do the unpleasant task by myself, but Virginia had been my nurse for so many months that I was spoiled. I liked having her take care of me.

One afternoon the dangling eyebrows needed cleaning and I called her in to help me. Immediately she got the Q-tips and the antiseptic solution and walked to my side. How many times she had leaned over to clean and probe and pull my face! I had marveled at her newfound strength. Before my crash she had been a fainter. The slightest sight of blood left her feeling weak. Years before on a camping vacation, our daughter Marlene had a mosquito bite become infected. We took her into a county emergency hospital to have the swelling checked by a doctor.

Virginia stood grimly by our daughter's side. Marlene was in tears. The doctor, out of sorts for being called from his golf game, lanced Marlene's swollen leg rather abruptly, and Virginia fainted away. Before the air crash, fainting had been her normal response to unpleasantness and pain. But for these past months she had worked with my bleeding face and hands without hesitation.

That day when she leaned over to clean my flopping eyebrows something amazing happened. She took one look at those pieces of hair and flesh and the room began to spin again. "I am going to faint, Merrill," she said and backed away. Her courage faded the moment my strength returned. I cleaned the eyebrows after that until Dr. Hamacher finally snipped them off. Both Virginia and I have wondered how she seemed to have endless personal resources as long as they were needed. When my strength returned, the sight of blood caused her to faint away again. When I was helpless—when I needed her—she was able to do anything. When my need passed, so did her courage.

There were other discoveries along the way. The doctors marveled that the intense heat of the crash and explosion had not blinded me. I retained my vision and didn't even need glasses. Still, my eyes caused many problems during those early surgeries. The eyelids that remained turned under at the extreme edges. The abrasive surfaces were scratching my eyeballs and creating ulcers on my eyes. To keep the lids from causing further damage, Dr. Hamacher had to reconstruct them. That meant sewing the outer eyelids together, leaving only a very small opening through which to see. With the eyelids turned under, I got ulcers on the eyeballs. With the eyelids sewed together, I could hardly see. Dr. Hamacher had to carefully rotate the skin flaps and suture them into place to get the eyelids to function again. He never did get back to making me new eyebrows.

The skin grafted across my mouth was tight and inflexible. To sing again with any kind of freedom meant rebuilding my mouth and lips. Virginia and Dr. Hamacher must have really enjoyed those early days of grafting around my mouth, because I couldn't speak to bother them and couldn't complain about anything.

My neck was forced down by scar tissue. The scars had to be removed and new split-thickness grafts from my chest had to be put on to release my neck and set my face free to move again.

In one surgery Dr. Hamacher removed sheets of skin from my hips and grafted it to my hands. That skin released the fingers from their claw position and let me play again. However, that same skin from my hips was never meant to take the abuse hands must take. In the sun my hands tan quickly. Except for white streaks on the surface, most of the skin of my hands appears almost black in the summertime. The skin on my face was not meant to be exposed to the weather changes, either. One afternoon I walked through a snowstorm in near-zero weather. My face felt like it was frostbitten. The sun does the same thing to it. My face and hands can feel any extreme weather change immediately.

All this skin that was being removed from my stomach or side or back left large raw areas. When they healed, especially the large donor areas on my stomach, they were hard and inflexible. At first I wondered if Dr. Hamacher was doing more damage to my unburned areas than he was helping to heal the burned ones. Then, over the years, the donor sites began to get soft again. Now, however, it is difficult to tell which areas were burned in the fire and which were scarred by the skin removed to be grafted elsewhere.

When I feel the discomfort from the scarred donor areas I think of that jacket I wore in the flames. How did it turn asbestoslike in the fire? How did that thin piece of artificial fabric protect the only areas where enough skin was available to rebuild my face and hands? What kept that fragile nylon shirt from bursting into flames? It is hard to feel ungrateful or complain about the donor-area scars, when it is those areas which

11

Handsome Is Something Inside

MY FACE HAS SHOCKED a lot of people. My picture has been used to scare reckless teenage drivers. One of my daughter's friends suggested I get work in Hollywood as a movie monster. Pedestrians passing me in the crosswalk have stopped in their tracks and begun walking backwards, staring at me, or gone around the block to see me again. I've seen children run to their parents in alarm as I approached them. Young people on the street call out to their friends, "Hey, look at that ugly man. Have you ever seen anything more ghastly?" I've seen people laugh and point as I pass. Drivers of cars next to mine have trouble keeping between the lines as they jockey for a place to stare at me as they drive.

I have responded in many different ways to those who stop and stare. I have responded in anger. One man in a restaurant stared at me continually for several minutes. Then he leaned over to the people at his table and had them stare at me. He laughed and pointed and discussed me for the length of his meal. He was not a handsome man himself, and when I finished eating, I walked over to his table and said angrily, "At least I wasn't born ugly." Then I turned and walked away.

I felt guilty about that for weeks. He had insulted and shamed me. But by returning the insult I was reduced to his level. And besides, if I saw someone like me pass by, I would stare, too. Hopefully I would stare with compassion, or catch myself staring and turn away immediately. Hopefully, if our eyes met before I turned away, I would smile and treat the person as another human being, with love and sympathetic respect. Now I expect people to stare at me. If they don't, I feel a bit left out. After all, if I saw me walking down the street somewhere, I would wonder what in the world happened to the poor guy!

At the first big convention I attended for the company after my accident, I was walking across the convention display area. People stared or smiled and walked away. I was a bit nervous because this was my first time back in public and I was there to sell the National Music Service to funeral directors at the convention. All of a sudden a woman fifty feet away yelled in my direction. "Hey, clown," she shouted, "take off your mask. It isn't Halloween yet." I looked up at her and for a moment our eyes met. When she saw I wasn't a clown in makeup, but a badly burned human being, she turned white with embarrassment. I walked up to her. She was frozen with fright and didn't even move. I said, "You didn't know what you were saying. It is all right."

She began to apologize. "Don't worry," I assured her. "It is an easy mistake to forgive. I was badly burned in a fire and the mask you see is my face. I can't take it off." We chatted there awhile and have seen each other since then on other convention display floors. Now she walks up to me and shakes my hand and recalls the horror that she felt that first moment she realized her mistake.

I was handsome before the accident. At least Virginia thought I was. Now everything was changed. But that doesn't mean I am ugly. I may look ugly, but I am not an ugly person. I often feel like fighting back when someone stares at me and says, "Look at that funny-looking guy. Look at that ugly man, the man with all the scars." I even get tense when people stare at me with sympathy or compassion. All I want is to be treated like a normal human being.

Actually, my new face has become a definite advantage. I am a salesman. I want to tell funeral directors about National Music

Service and the advantages our system has over the competition. But at every convention there are competitors who want to do the same thing. There are many companies competing for the same market. Their salesmen come in all shapes and sizes. But in comparison to my face, they all look alike. I don't need a business card. Nobody forgets my face. That is a real advantage.

Perhaps that is my way of rationalizing all the pain and suffering. But to be driven into a shell—to lock myself in a closet because people stare at me—would be to give up and die. Sure, there are bad times. I especially hate it when people look at me with pity in their eyes. I have a little conversation with myself at times like that. I say, "Don't feel sorry for me, buddy. I am alive and well. I have a wonderful business and I do what I like doing best. God has given me a song and I am singing it."

After that stage in my private inner dialogue to remind myself of my blessing, I may feel like saying, "What about your life, buddy? You have a face without scars, but what about the scars in your soul? What about your life? Are you happy? Are you doing what you want to do? Are you alive and well with a wife and family that loves you? Do you have a song and are you singing it?"

I suppose this private conversation shouldn't be necessary, but I am surrounded by people who feel that scars and handicaps and suffering are to be avoided at all costs. People tell me that they couldn't possibly love a God who had anything to do with such a tragedy as mine. And I have to respond to them with, "Don't call it a tragedy. My experience has led to all kinds of growth for me and my family. Don't make judgments on the surface appearances. Go below the surface and see what's happening there." I really believe that most of the people who pass me on the street don't understand at all. If they knew the kind of life I have, I honestly believe they would envy me.

My face has also become a source of wonderful humor. On my

first business trip by commercial jet from Spokane to Los Angeles, I sat next to a businessman who took one look at me and wanted desperately to ask about my scars. Finally, as we were taking off down the runway, he turned to me and blurted out, "What in the devil happened to you?"

I thought to myself that this was a most unfortunate moment to answer his question. However, since he asked, I turned to him and smiled through the scars. My eyes were sealed almost closed. I still had no nose, no eyebrows, and little stubby ears. "I had an airplane crash." For an instant the man stared at me. The plane began to leave the ground. Suddenly the man stiffened in his seat. His legs shot out and his hands gripped the seat belt. He remained that way the entire trip to Los Angeles. And when we finally landed safely he breathed a sigh of relief I will never forget.

*   *   *   *   *

BEING STARED AT HAS become a kind of adventure for Merrill. But the family and I have had real trouble with it from the start. When his face was almost sealed closed and he could only see out of a portion of one eye, people stared so often and so long that the rest of us could hardly stand it. Merrill was too busy struggling to see to notice how impolite and rude some people would be. In restaurants the children would take it so long and then look up at me as if to say, "Mom, see that guy staring at Daddy. I would like to walk right over to that man and hit him in the nose." We all wanted to defend Merrill. We hated the way people stared or walked backward or rolled down their windows for a better look. He was my husband. He was their father. And we loved him. Still people stared. Finally we decided that people stare at celebrities, too. We would pretend he was a celebrity. We would make their stares into compliments. And sometimes it worked.

People were staring and laughing at the man I married and it made me mad. He was very handsome when we met. He had thick, curly hair and a wonderful, winsome grin. He had a dimple in his chin and his skin was soft and smooth. He was strong and athletic. His hands were fun to hold. His lips were round and smooth, and I loved to kiss them. I found him very attractive. Then suddenly all was changed.

Every time he came home from surgery he looked different. His skin was hard and bumpy. His lips were gone. His hair was burned away. It was difficult for him to breathe through his new nostrils without making little gasping sounds. His hands felt strange to touch. His face was often hard for a long time after surgery. The man I married was still inside, but the man outside had changed. And though I was in love with the man inside Merrill, I also loved the man outside. That man was gone, and the man in his place didn't kiss like the other man would kiss. His skin felt different from the other man's skin. And at first it was a problem to me. I made up my mind that whatever he looked like didn't matter. I loved him before the crash. I would love him after. But there were times I stared at his old pictures and longed to have the outside Merrill back again.

Time passed. We solved a lot of problems together. I watched my husband laughing and singing and struggling. I felt his arms around me. I felt him kissing me again. I began to see familiar old expressions in the unfamiliar face. I began to see his eyes flashing love across the room at me as they did before the accident. I was falling in love again with the same man, even though he didn't look the same—because I was in love with what he was, not with what he looked like. I was having a romance with the brave, determined man I married. And in my eyes he got more and more handsome every day.

Surgery after surgery, I saw his new face emerge. After all, that new face was partly my creation. All those scabs I had pulled off, all that slime I had cleaned away, and all that pain and suffering

had been for this moment. Out of the ashes of a burned marshmallow swollen big as a basketball, charcoal-black, wrinkled and
bleeding, emerged a handsome man. Dr. Hamacher was building
a fine new face, and when people stared I found it difficult to
understand why Merrill wasn't as handsome to them as he was to
me. He may not have eyebrows and eyelashes. He may have
rough, uneven skin, but his new face was handsome. Still they
stared and pointed and laughed.

Little by little it dawned on me what "handsome" is. Handsome is knowing the person behind the face. Handsome is something inside that person shining out through him. Handsome
isn't what a person looks like. It is what a person is. And Merrill
is the most handsome man I know.

* * * * *

I NEVER FELT UGLY even when I looked in the mirror. So people
who found me ugly or strange were always a surprise to me.
Virginia and I went to New York for a national television show
four or five years ago. I thought I looked fairly decent then, but
the people had invited me because they had heard me sing before
the accident. They had not seen me since. They had heard records but had no idea of my burns or plastic surgery.

When we arrived at the studio, an assistant to the producer met
us and escorted us to a little waiting room. We sat there for over
an hour before I realized they didn't know what to do with me.
Virginia and I decided it was their problem and we would wait to
see how well they handled it. Finally the producer himself
knocked on the door.

"Come in," I answered.

The producer stood there looking down at me. He whistled
softly to himself and sat down beside me on the sofa.

"Merrill," he said, "we have a problem."

"Oh, really!" I pretended surprise. "What is that?"

For a moment he sat in stunned silence. I knew what his problem was and I couldn't wait to see him solve it. Finally he got honest.

"We don't know what to do with you. All our viewers will see your burns and wonder what happened. We just wanted you to sing. Now you will have to talk as well."

When the cameras were turned on and the program began, the host introduced us to his audience and we spent almost the entire time talking about my accident. I suppose they were embarrassed and wanted me to explain. It was a very disappointing moment. To think how much our faces get in each other's way. I think everyone on that program would have been grateful if I had called and canceled my appearance on that show because I looked different. But you can't stop living because you are scarred or deformed or handicapped. You can't just quit because you cause people embarrassment or discomfort.

Several years ago I met a man who was injured in a helicopter crash. He had been wearing a helmet and so he was only burned from his eyebrows down to his chin. After the surgery he never left his home. He had his food brought in to him. His wife and family had to leave him because he was constantly depressed. He didn't want to see or talk to anyone. He sat in his room, locked behind his front door. He brooded over what might have been and was angry and embarrassed because of his scars. So I drove down to see him.

He let me in the door and sat there looking angry. I began to share what had happened to me and why I refused to give in to all the stares and taunts, but the more I talked, the angrier he became. I tried to be polite, but he wouldn't listen. So I yelled at him, "Go ahead, sit here and die if you want to. But don't forget you can go out into the world and be useful again. You can laugh and love and live again, if you'll just try." He kicked me out of his house.

How many times Dr. Hamacher told me about patients who got little scars and went home to die. "God has given them the gift of life," he mused, "and they go home and waste it." Several weeks later in the Portland International Airport, I saw the man who kicked me out of his house. He was wearing a new suit and carrying a briefcase. When he saw me he came running through the crowds yelling, "Merrill, you were right." We embraced. There we stood, the burned and scarred "abnormals" in the middle of a crowd of "normals," and all of them staring at us. Arm in arm we walked through that crowd. Words tumbled out of him, about his family and his new job. "I decided," he said, "you were right. It was time to get out and be useful again." Many people were staring now, and we could feel their stares. He waved and started to walk away. Suddenly he turned and winked at me, lifting one thumb high in the pilot's signal that all is well. Then he disappeared into the crowd. People still stared and pointed as I walked back to my gate. They had no idea why I was crying. It wasn't for the scars I carried, but because one scarred young man was alive again.

Some never get over their scars. My father never got over mine. He wanted to protect me from further accidents. He wanted me to slow down and take it easy. He begged me not to work so hard. He scolded me for traveling around the country again. And above all else, he hated to see me fly again.

I loved my father. I did not want to hurt him, but I had to fly. I loved flying and it was important to my business that we get about the country quickly and economically. So I bought a new plane and began to fly again. A year and a half later Dad went out to roll up his car windows, had a heart attack, and died. He was only sixty-one. I know he never got over that first look he had at me lying in the ambulance. That, and worrying about it happening again, led to his death. Still I could not stop flying out of fear—his or mine. I could not change my entire life because of what might happen. He had to let me go and he could not.

Now that my own children are grown and have families of their own, I understand better what agony it is to let them go. Now I know better why he insisted on the family gathering for that Thanksgiving feast each year. Now I know how it feels to want my children around me. I want to love and protect them. I don't want them to suffer the way I suffered; yet I must let them go. I must let them take charge of their own lives even if in the process they suffer.

12

Through Christ Who Strengthens Me

THE PORTLAND CIVIC AUDITORIUM was filling rapidly with excited young people who had come in busloads from all over northern Oregon. Merrill was scheduled to sing in twenty minutes, and already most of the seats were filled. I entered the auditorium, walked down a side aisle, and sat near the stage. Finally the preliminary program ended and the emcee stood to introduce my husband. He spoke of Merrill's ordeal as one of "faith and testing few men survive." Then the orchestra began to play. Merrill walked onto the stage and into a bright pool of light. As he sang, my head was filled with memories.

It was hard to believe that those little children who clustered around me in the kitchen Thanksgiving Day thirteen years ago were all grown now. Judie, Marlene, and Dan were married, with homes and families of their own. It was hard to believe that the handsome man I married could survive a flaming crash though ugly, burned, and bleeding, and now wear a strange new face and hands. It is hard to believe that the fainting housewife who wondered before the accident if she was really needed, could pull scabs, change messy sheets and make important decisions about air ambulances, burn wards, and plastic surgeons. But most of all, it was hard to believe that any of it ever really happened.

There he was, up on the stage singing as he had always sung. Our plane was parked at Portland's International Airport. We had flown over Beaver Marsh that day and didn't even think to look down into those trees where the wreckage still lay untouched after all these years. How did we get through those painful, lonely hours? What pulled us through the endless days of treatment and surgery, the long, restless, dream-tossed nights? How did we get here from there?

As Merrill sang, I remembered our daughter Judie. When she was just a baby we would take her to our little office where we sometimes worked until late at night. She would play contentedly for a while, then lie down where she was playing and go to sleep. One morning, about two o'clock, we found Judie curled up in a little ball, lying on top of a stereo-speaker box, a twelve-inch cube, sound asleep. We picked her up, put her in the car, and returned home. When Judie awakened the next morning she asked, "How did I get here?" She was home, but she didn't remember how she got there from the office.

Those past years had been like that for me. I remember driving through a blizzard to Klamath Falls, but after that it was all kind of blurry. At the concert that night I asked myself, "How did I get here from there?" And I thought of Judie going to sleep confident that her parents would get her through the night. Merrill and I had been delivered through the night by our Heavenly Father. I doubt we could have made it without Him. That verse I recalled one night in a Klamath Falls motel room—"I can do all things through Christ who strengthens me"—had been proven true.

Now I watched my husband on that stage. I had grown to love his new face with all its bumps and scars. Perhaps it seems a rationalization to others, but the family and I thought him more handsome than before. As he sang that night, my heart almost burst with love for him. But at the same time I felt a strange old feeling in my stomach. The audience was applauding for encores. Merrill was singing and sharing, and somehow I felt alone again. I had hardly seen him in the past few months. He was traveling up and down the country, performing at conventions and in large concert halls. He was busy representing National Music Service at important meetings and at individual funeral homes. Coordinating sales, services, and new-product development for a multimillion-dollar company meant that Merrill needed to be on the road again. There were no more scabs to pull, no more oozing sores to dress, no more emergency decisions to make. The children were gone and I was alone in an empty house. I knew Merrill loved me, but the old feelings of worthlessness were coming to life in me again.

The audience was standing now and applauding for one final encore. Merrill began to sing: "Amazing grace—how sweet the sound. . . ." Though I was grateful to God for getting us through those past years, I felt strangely angry and disappointed that they were over. I know it sounds awful, but I had found purpose through Merrill's crash and hospitalization. My husband had needed me. I had been an intimate part of his life. For long months he lay helpless, blind, bleeding—and I had nursed him through. During the years of surgery and recuperation, we had spent hours together talking about everything and everybody. We had laughed and cried and suffered together. Now I almost had to make an appointment to see him. He was often gone for weeks at a time, and even when we talked, I sensed that other things were on his mind.

At first I could handle being alone again. I could call Judie or Marlene or Dan. I could baby-sit the grandchildren. I could putter around our offices. But the children really didn't need me anymore and the office took care of itself. Where once I had been secretary, office manager, bookkeeper and handyman, now dozens of employees scurried about. I felt I was in their way. I tried becoming a faithful housewife again, but the house was empty and there was seldom anyone to cook or clean for.

As my depression worsened, I felt guilty. "What kind of person are you?" I would scold myself. "Look at all the wonderful things you have!"—"So what good is a beautiful home and nice clothes and a savings account when you feel alone and worthless?" I answered. "What good is it to have everything you want except a reason to live?" At the lowest moment in my growing depression I even wondered about ending my own life.

Merrill was still up there singing as memories tumbled in my mind. "Through many dangers, toils, and snares, I have already come. . . ." He sang it and it was true. But past victories did not guarantee future ones. As my depression grew, I had finally decided to see a professional Christian counselor. Going to a professional and paying him to listen to my problems was a frightening and embarrassing new experience for me. I remember driving to his office at least an hour early and sitting in the car, hoping no one who knew me would see me there. I was ashamed and afraid. I did not want anyone to think that Merrill Womach's wife would have problems. He was so strong, so full of faith. What would they think if they saw me going to a counselor? What if they knew how weak my faith was—even after all I had seen God do for us?

Minutes before my scheduled appointment time I hurried into his office and buried myself behind a magazine in the waiting room. "Christians don't have problems," I thought to myself. "What are you doing here?"—"But Christians do have problems," I argued back, "and I am here to let God help me solve them through this trained and gifted person."

Since that first visit, I have learned many things about myself and God's plan for my life. I have also learned not to be ashamed of my need to seek help. The counseling I received was an important step used by God in rebuilding my life.

As I sat in the Civic Auditorium, reliving that first visit, I heard my name being called. "Virginia," Merrill said, "please stand so these people can see you." He was pointing at me from the stage at the Portland Civic Auditorium. The crowd applauded for me, and Merrill began to speak.

"You are looking at a strong, brave person," he told them. "For the past years she has been my nurse, my counselor, my closest friend, and my wife. She cared for my burned face when no one else wanted to touch it. She wiped slime from my fingers and cried tears of joy when I played again. She helped me up when my legs wobbled and she walked the house with me when nightmares of burning flesh kept me awake. Virginia, I love you," he said, "and I am forever grateful for what you were and are to me."

Then they applauded again. And Merrill smiled down at me through his tears. The houselights came on and he was surrounded by a crowd of friends and admirers. I sat there in the auditorium watching him reach out to all those dear young people. I could tell that the time with him had made a great deal of difference in their lives. They had heard through his new lips how God had helped him survive the suffering. And as they listened to Merrill sing and share his faith, each of them grew stronger, more able to face the suffering in his own life.

I was glad and proud and grateful that night, but I still felt lonely. This was the beginning of another new period in our lives. God had given Merrill a song and he had to sing it. That meant jetting across the continent, with hotel rooms and restaurant meals for him. But what did it mean for me? I could travel with Merrill; he had really made that clear, and I would. But maybe God had a song for me to sing. In my counseling I was learning again that I, too, was a person who had gifts. I had a contribution to make. I, too, had responsibilities to my family, to my God, to my marriage.

So the hospital period in our lives was over. We could work out a new-style partnership for the new kind of life that lay ahead. Those days in the hospital and in our home, when Merrill and I shared twenty-four-hour intimacy, were gone. And the shock of that change had gotten to me, but I learned in that Klamath Falls emergency hospital that I did not have to faint away because my life had changed. I could stand and face that tragedy. If I could pick off scabs with a tweezers and if I could dress those burns, I could do anything.

Now my new work was cut out for me. I had to help us build a relationship that would weather all the travel and the changes that lay ahead. I had to set some new goals for myself. I had to find new ways to invest my gifts and energy. And I had to speak up for my rights as a wife and still help Merrill sing his song.

The auditorium was almost empty now. Merrill walked over to me and reached out his hands. "Let's go home, honey," he said. I grabbed his hands, now clean and strong again, and we embraced. Then we walked up that long, slanting aisle together and in my heart I knew, "I can do all things through Christ who strengthens me."

*   *   *   *   *

SOMETIME JUST BEFORE the crash, I had been invited to sing at another large interchurch youth rally in Tacoma, Washington. It wasn't easy to be on the road all the time. It wasn't easy to sleep in motels, eat in restaurants, and live out of a suitcase. That day in Tacoma, I was sick of it. I had accepted their invitation months before, and the sponsors of the concert had advertised widely and rented the largest auditorium in their city. They were depending on me, and I was only there because I felt I had no other choice.

I called Virginia and shared my loneliness. Then I talked to each of the children. Sometimes that's a remedy for homesickness, but this time it just made me feel all the worse. So I left the motel and began to walk. "What is it," I wondered to myself, "that makes me what I am? Why is it so hard to change? I have always been a fighter, a man on the go. I have always worked too hard, expected too much from myself and those around me, and tried to cram too much into each new day."

I turned into a little park and watched the children playing. "Why am I on the road away from my wife and children when I could be at home with them around the fireplace enjoying a normal kind of family life?" We have a great family and we have wonderful times together, but there has never been enough time to do everything I wanted to do. I loved the idea of building National Music Service into a strong company serving thousands of funeral homes across America. I loved the idea of using stereo cassettes to minister to the bereaved in hundreds of different places all at once. I loved singing to people in concerts and sharing my faith with an auditorium filled with teenagers and adults. I loved being with my family eating watermelon in our backyard or sailing together on the lake. I loved it all. But that night in Tacoma it was getting to me. "I do not have to sing tonight," I thought. "I will just call them and tell them I have decided to return at once. Then I will drive to the airport and fly home. I will break this cycle. I will work only forty or fifty hours a week and spend the rest of the time with my family. I will park my plane, unpack my suitcase, hang up my garment bag, and forget it for a while."

I walked back toward the motel room and watched a Little League team practicing nearby. As I stood staring at the players through the wire fence, I knew that the idea of canceling my schedule for the next few weeks or months was a pipe dream. I knew I could not stop. Early in my life something set the pace in me, and I had been on the go ever since.

When I was in the fifth grade I wanted to play baseball, but the coach at Bryant Elementary School wouldn't let me play on the team. He said I was too small. Instead of getting discouraged about it, I answered, "Okay, fine." Then I went down to a local city park that had a baseball field and asked the grounds keeper if I could rent the ball park. He laughed at me but we struck up a bargain. He said he would rent the baseball field to me for five cents a game. Over the next few weeks, I organized twelve teams in the city grade schools. These weren't softball teams like we had in grade school. These were hardball teams, and we played in a real baseball park. We even got the mothers to make rough but colorful uniforms. The other kids flocked to join. The poor old coach didn't have anybody at Bryant Elementary to make up a team anymore, and he finally gave in and offered to coach our league if we would play on the school grounds.

I've always been that way, doing a dozen things at once. My dad would ask, "What are you trying to do? Why are you in such a hurry? Slow down!"

As I dressed for that concert years ago I felt confused and tired —to get up in front of all those people and sing for the next two hours seemed a grim, impossible task. Just then I heard a timid knock on my door. A young man stood there looking bashful and embarrassed.

"Excuse me, Mr. Womach," he said. "Do you mind if we talk for a moment?"

"No," I replied, "come in while I finish dressing." The young man was in his early twenties. He sat down and began speaking rather quietly.

"Do you remember when you sang here three years ago at the Voice of Christian Youth rally?"

"Yes, I remember. Why?"

"Well," he hesitated, "when you invited people in the audience to accept Christ as Lord of their lives, I did not respond to your invitation to believe in any way, but I went home and your words and songs really stuck with me. That night I became a Christian and I just wanted you to know."

We talked for a while and then he excused himself. I quickly finished dressing and hurried to the concert. Backstage the director asked if a young man had spoken to me in my room earlier. When I responded affirmatively, he told me there was a sequel to the story. The young man was then in seminary, studying for the ministry. Already the director knew of twenty-four other young people that young man had led to Christ since his decision the night of my concert three years before.

I heard the orchestra play and stepped out to begin my concert. I sang for an hour and then returned to my room. I could feel that young man's presence there. As I lay in that motel bed, I couldn't help but pray: "God, I complained I didn't really want to sing in Tacoma either of those evenings. I really didn't see much purpose in being there. I felt that I was just entertaining people and not doing very much. Then You sent this young man to remind me that You are at work in my life. Forgive me."

Before that night was over, I got out of bed and knelt beside it. I wanted to show God that I was serious when I prayed: "Lord, whatever it takes, and I don't care what it is, use me. Do whatever You have to do to me, but use me."

Several days later my plane crashed into the woods at Beaver Marsh. Some people may recoil at this. They might shout at me, "Are you saying your God burned you on purpose? What kind of God is that?"

I wish I could crack open that mystery. I wish I could say exactly how God works. But I know one thing: Although I did not like the pain and the suffering or the disfigurement, I am convinced beyond a shadow of a doubt that the effectiveness of my life in Christ, the growth of my business, and the opportunities I have to sing and share my faith around the world have multiplied a hundred times since that crash. I don't like people staring at me. I am human. I have feelings. But if you said, "Merrill, do you want to be the way you were before?" I would say, "No, I want to be the way God wants me to be. And because I believe that this is what God wants, I pray now, as I prayed in that hotel room in Tacoma, *Whatever it takes, Lord, use me.*

13

Something Beautiful

THIRTEEN YEARS AFTER that flaming crash, once again my plane circled the emergency landing field at Beaver Marsh, Oregon. A camera crew and I were searching for the remaining wreckage in the dense woods down below. Months before, documentary filmmaker, Mel White, had approached me about doing a film on my crash and the ensuing years of plastic surgery. I had not been interested in doing a film before. I could not see anything about our lives that would be particularly significant or meaningful. Then I watched two other films he had recently produced—on the practical side of Christian faith. *Though I Walk Through the Valley* documents the last six months in the life of a terminal cancer patient and his family. It demonstrates the power of God to help man face death and dying. *In the Presence of Mine Enemies* is a documentary on the life of an American prisoner of war and the seven and a half years of separation from his wife and family in a jungle prison solitary-confinement cell. It was another incredible testimony to the power of God to help us survive those inevitable tragic times. Mel proposed a third film to feature Virginia and me called *He Restoreth My Soul.* This film would also use a theme from the Twenty-third Psalm and would document the part God played in restoring our inner lives, while the doctors tried to restore my face and hands. We agreed to the project and now we were flying to the place where it all began.

We couldn't see the wreckage from the air, and after landing hiked into the forest in the general direction of the crash site. It wasn't long before we spotted it—a tangle of rusted airplane parts, burned recording equipment, and fallen trees. The sun was shining. The air was warm. There was no snow on the ground, but I could still feel that snow cascading down off the loaded limbs onto my burning face. I could still feel the pain and see the ball of flame that almost consumed me.

"Get a microphone on Merrill," the director instructed sound-man Fred Roberts. Dan Dunkelberger, the cameraman, had already loaded the portable sound camera and walked slowly in front of me as I approached the wreckage.

"Action! Merrill, describe the wreck. How did you feel as the plane tumbled through the trees?"

I could hear my own voice describing those split seconds of terror before I lost consciousness. I pointed to the still-scarred trees that had whipped the plane around and sent it crashing backwards to the ground in flames. But as I stood in the wreckage holding pieces of steel fused together by the intensity of that fire, I thought of God and wondered at the role He played in all of this. In those few minutes between the explosion and my escape, amazing things had taken place. I tore in half a five-hundred-pound-test seat belt. I forced open the mangled, twisted door with hands already burned away. My entire body was burned except for an area covered by a synthetic jacket hardened in the flames—which protected the only skin areas adequate to graft my other burns. My lungs and vocal cords had been protected by a small layer of air from the fire that fused steel and charred and twisted the entire fuselage. And I sang all the way to the hospital, and thus avoided the shock which is a primary killer of serious burn victims.

What could I say? That God planned the crash down to each minute detail? Or that my careless oversight caused the crash, and He intervened to save me? What difference does it make, when you are confident that God is alive and working in your life to accomplish your good? I stood in the wreckage that day. The cameras rolled as I sang of God's perfect peace in times of tragedy and suffering. And as I sang, I realized again—what would our lives be without Him?

* * * * *

I DIDN'T FLY TO Beaver Marsh that day with Merrill and the crew. The sight of that wreckage would have been too painful for me, I'm afraid. The next day they interviewed me sitting on the edge of my bed in our home in Spokane. It was the first time anyone had asked me how I felt during those horrible hours on Thanksgiving Day. I could not control the tears as I remembered that first awful look at the man on the bed with the giant, burned head.

Merrill suffered terribly. I hated his pain. There was no pleasure in picking off his scabs or changing his bloody sheets, either. The whole family suffered. It would be a lie to say that this was an enjoyable or easy experience. It was not. And I would not want to go through it again, but I do not believe it was a tragic accident without purpose or meaning.

People often ask if I believe that God burned Merrill. I don't think He did. God *allowed* Merrill to go through this tragedy. Merrill was like Job, in a way. God didn't make Job go through his tragedies either. God allowed Job to experience them for a purpose, but God spared Job's life. God spared Merrill's life, as well. He allowed Merrill to go through the fire. He had a special reason for what we have been through together. I don't believe it was an accident. I think God chose our family to go through this. And although it sounds strange, I feel it is an honor that He chose us. God had a purpose in all our suffering, and I believe it is to share the strength we have gained from it with others who have suffered or who will suffer tragedy in their lives.

The next afternoon they filmed an interview with Merrill and Dr. Hamacher in the operating room where Merrill had more than fifty surgeries. Merrill sat bare-chested on the edge of the operating table. As the camera crew put the microphone around

Hamacher's neck, I heard him joking with Merrill about the extra weight around my husband's waistline. Merrill pointed at the doctor's wide girth, and they both laughed and teased each other mercilessly. I could smell Dr. Hamacher's cigar hidden somewhere in a nearby ashtray, and I remembered how often that smell had signalled his caring presence in our lives.

He had been our doctor, but more important, he had been our friend. He made it clear to me that family support could make the difference in Merrill's recovery. He called a meeting of our wider family and set the ground rules to make us "a recovery team," instead of "an advice-giving, patient-confusing, doctor-baiting, nurse-infuriating, hospital-interfering" family unit that well-meaning but uninformed families can become. He laid down the line about painkilling drugs and scrupulously prevented Merrill from becoming a hospital-produced drug addict. He brought humor, honesty, confrontation, and love to our family. And when we got his major bill, which included those first ten weeks of constant care, at least six major surgeries (one of them six hours in length), and visits usually twice a day including Sundays, he charged us only $575.00. Then, because we had so little income then, he let us charge our bills for two years without payment.

Hamacher is not a pious man, but a man of deep personal conviction. During the interview as he recalled those years of work on Merrill's face and hands, he turned to the camera and reminisced. "Throughout all of these years of painful suffering," he said, "Merrill never stopped believing in God, and that can make a tremendous difference for any family mixed up in a major catastrophe like this one."

*   *   *   *   *

THE VETERANS HOSPITAL in Spokane has hundreds of men and women who are suffering from painful burns and a variety of other maladies. Virginia and I entered the large ward where the camera crew was setting up. Dozens of patients sat waiting for my concert. Some were missing an arm or a leg. Others had burns wrapped in gauze. Several were immobilized in traction with broken bones. Others sat in quiet shock, recuperating from wounds that went far deeper than a burn or break.

The director signalled the camera to roll.

"Fellows," I began, "fourteen years ago if I had stood here before you I would not have understood what you are going through. But in the past fourteen years I have suffered. My face and hands were burned off in a flaming air crash. You can see from these scars how much the doctors have done to restore my physical body. But the history of those painful years would not impress you. You are here today and you are suffering, too. You know what pain feels like. You have learned that pain is a fact of life. They can give you drugs for pain. Doctors and nurses have needles and pills to help get you through the physical suffering. But what about the pain inside you that comes from loneliness or fear? They can't give you enough shots or pills to take that pain away. Only God can help you bear that kind of pain. You are not alone. He is with you! When you feel lonely call out to Him. He will hear you and help you. When you are afraid, reach out and He will take your hand."

What more could I say? You can't make a person believe. You can't convince him there is a God or that God can be a real help in troubled times. You can only say, "When you are suffering, reach out and you will find Him there!" Then I began to sing the film's theme song. The words were perfect and told my story well:

Happy Again

I've been happy before,
I'll be happy again.
There'll be rainbows
To fill the sky and silver linings again.

He has promised to dry
Ev'ry tear from my eye.
I will trust Him today,
Though skies are gray, I'll be happy again.

There was music before,
There'll be music again.
There's a song in my heart
He did impart, I'll sing it again.

Through the dark lonely night,
He will guide me and then,
I will look in His face,
Amazing grace, I'll be happy again.

There was someone before,
There'll be someone again,
Even death cannot conquer
Now, His grave is empty, my friend.

When the dark billows roll,
He restoreth my soul.
Though there's trouble today
I hear Him say, you'll be happy again.

Though there's trouble today
I hear Him say, you'll be happy again.

When the singing and the sharing ended, we walked around
the ward from bed to bed. One old man took my hand and began
to cry, but he was smiling through the tears. He understood.
Others looked angry and abandoned. If only they could see that
anger is a dead end. If only they could see that suffering can be

God's way of leading us to Him. A mother goes through suffering to have a baby. She doesn't like the pain or the inconvenience of those nine long months. But when the child is born, the mother forgets the pain and rejoices in this new life. For me, suffering was the way to something new in our lives—and though I hated the pain, I would go through it again.

As we turned to leave, one of the nurses who had heard the concert in the hospital ward came up to me. She had stood outside in the hall as I sang and shared. As we were leaving she spoke to me.

"Mr. Womach," she said, "I am sorry for what happened to you."

She missed the whole point. Nobody needs to feel sorry for me. This past experience has been beautiful. I did not like the pain. I yelled for painkillers like everybody else, but the pain was taking me somewhere. I tried to tell her again that God has a plan to develop us. My suffering had a purpose. She shook her head and feigned a smile, but I knew she didn't understand.

"Don't be afraid of suffering," I told her. "God is in that, too!"

*   *   *   *   *

ONE YOUNG MAN UNDERSTOOD Merrill when he spoke that way. He was a sculptor, and after hearing Merrill share his experiences in a luncheon club, the young man went to Beaver Marsh, found the airplane wreckage and carted a trunkload home to his studio. There he shaped from the worthless, rusted metal a five-foot-high assemblage of Christ on the cross.

He called us one morning, introduced himself and presented his assemblage to Merrill. We had no idea what he had made, but our staff gathered around the young man who stood before a tall, incredibly beautiful statue. Christ was there. His arms were pieces of the charred fuselage. His chest was made of rusty springs from the pilot's seat found in the wreckage. His face was a gauge from the cockpit. In some incredible way the artist captured our Lord's suffering with a pile of wreckage. The young artist spoke words that described perfectly how Merrill and I still feel.

"When Christ died on the cross two thousand years ago," he said, "His disciples were shocked and disappointed. 'What a terrible thing for this man to suffer and die,' they thought. 'What a useless, horrible waste.' Then, out of the suffering emerged God's greatest gift to man, a way of salvation. Out of death came new life. Out of suffering came joy. This assemblage is a symbol. By turning pieces of old wreckage into something beautiful, I wanted to show what God has done in the lives of Merrill and Virginia. They have suffered. But God has shaped their suffering into something beautiful."

   As the young man spoke, Merrill reached out and took my hand. I looked into his eyes. We both were crying. Fourteen years of pain and suffering flowed between us through tightly clasped hands. That young sculptor understood. God had tested us by fire. And out of the suffering—He was making something beautiful in our lives.